Obesity

HUMAN DEVELOPMENT PERSPECTIVES

Obesity
Health and Economic Consequences of an Impending Global Challenge

Meera Shekar and Barry Popkin, Editors

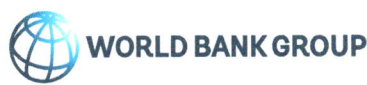
WORLD BANK GROUP

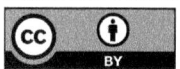

Human Development Perspectives

The books in this series address main and emerging development issues of a global/regional nature through original research and findings in the areas of education, gender, health, nutrition, population, and social protection and jobs. The series is aimed at policy makers and area experts and is overseen by the Human Development Practice Group Chief Economist.

Previous titles in this series

Truman Packard, Ugo Gentilini, Margaret Grosh, Philip O'Keefe, Robert Palacios, David Robalino, and Indhira Santos, *Protecting All: Risk Sharing for a Diverse and Diversifying World of Work* (2019).

Damien de Walque, *Risking Your Health: Causes, Consequences, and Interventions to Prevent Risky Behaviors* (2014).

Rita Almeida, Jere Behrman, and David Robalino, *The Right Skills for the Job? Rethinking Training Policies for Workers* (2012).

Barbara Bruns, Deon Filmer, and Harry Anthony Patrinos, *Making Schools Work: New Evidence on Accountability Reforms* (2011).

Harold Alderman, *No Small Matter: The Impact of Poverty, Shocks, and Human Capital Investments in Early Childhood Development* (2011).

All books in the Human Development Perspectives series are available at https://openknowledge.worldbank.org/handle/10986/2161.

Contents

Boxes

Maps

Tables

Foreword

Being overweight/obese has long been perceived to be a problem only in high-income countries. However, recent data show that since 1975 obesity has nearly tripled and it now accounts for 4 million deaths globally every year. In 2016, over 2 billion people globally (44 percent) were overweight or obese, and more than 70 percent of these live in low- or middle-income countries, dispelling the myth that obesity is a problem only in high-income countries. Further, somewhat unexpectedly, 55 percent of the global rise of obesity is in rural areas, highlighting the huge potential negative economic and health impacts, especially for the poor and people living in rural areas. Overweight/obesity has a large impact on national economies—through reduced productivity, increased disability, increased health care costs, and reduced life expectancy. For example, in China between 2000 and 2009, the estimates of increased health care costs associated with obesity grew from 0.56 percent to 3.13 percent of China's annual national health care expenditure. In Brazil, obesity-related health care costs are expected to double, from US$5.8 billion in 2010 to US$10.1 billion in 2050.

Today, overweight/obesity-related non-communicable diseases are among the top-three killers in every region of the world except Sub-Saharan Africa. Furthermore, as obesity increases rapidly and child stunting rates decline at relatively slow rates, many countries across the globe are now suffering from what is referred to as the "double burden of malnutrition"—high stunting and increasing obesity rates—thereby further jeopardizing human capital.

This report, *Obesity: Health and Economic Consequences of an Impending Global Challenge*, is timely as it complements some recent and forthcoming technical reports on this issue. It is also at the core of the World Bank's Human Capital Project, which highlights the importance of investing in people to boost economic growth. The report reviews the changing epidemiology of overweight/obesity; current trends globally and by region, gender, and age; the health and economic costs and the potential impacts of failure to address it, including the impact on the climate; the potential effectiveness of policies and interventions; and country experiences and lessons learned, particularly with diet-related taxes and other preventive actions across several sectors. It puts forward a call to action for next steps in fighting this growing challenge.

Reducing overweight/obesity is a global public good. While the evidence base is still emerging, many countries are already struggling to put in place new policies, such as taxation on unhealthy foods and interpretive front-of-package labels, to urgently address this looming epidemic. Governments and development partners such as the World Bank have key roles to play in supporting this effort through a transformative approach and additional financial and human resources dedicated to this agenda. Scaling up promising interventions and policies, supporting reforms through multisectoral engagement, including through the private sector, and continuing to build the evidence base are key to preventing the rise of overweight/obesity in future generations. Proactively addressing this issue will contribute significantly to building human capital, ensuring higher economic growth, and sustaining a workforce that is healthy and prepared for a productive future.

Annette Dixon
Vice President, Human Development
World Bank

Acknowledgments

This report was prepared by a team led by Meera Shekar (World Bank), who conceptualized the overall report, co-authored several chapters, and provided guidance and direction for the report. Barry Popkin (UNC Chapel Hill), Julia Dayton Eberwein (Consultant), and Anne Marie Provo and Kyoko Shibata Okamura (World Bank) contributed substantially to the overall report, as well as to several chapters. Pia Schneider, Jonathan Kweku Akuoku, Georges Bianco Darido (World Bank), and Vanessa Oddo (Consultant) contributed as co-authors for specific chapters.

Anne Marie Provo and Carolyn Shelton led consultations with several World Bank sectoral teams. Juan Pablo Orjuela (Consultant), and Felipe Targa and Georges Bianco Darido from the World Bank's Transport Global Practice (GP) contributed to chapter 5.

The team is grateful to Maria Eugenia Bonilla-Chacin for initiating and managing the country case studies with guidance from the Global Delivery Initiative (GDI) team. The authors also acknowledge the country case study authors, who include Ana Carolina Feldenheimer da Silva (Brazil), Ariel Azar Denecken (Chile), Arun Nair (Kerala state, India), Mireya Vilar Compte (Mexico), Michal Brzezinski (Poland), Zandile Mchiza (South Africa), Nimal Weerasinghe (Sri Lanka), Sueppong Gowachirapant (Thailand), Sutayut Osornprasop (Thailand), Sirinya Phulkerd (Thailand), and Safir Sumer (Turkey).

Task Team Leaders for the country case studies include Daniela Pena de Lima (Brazil), Linda Brooke Schultz (Chile), Suresh Kunhi Mohammed (Kerala state, India), Claudia Macias (Mexico), Jakub Jan Kakietek (Poland), Anna Koziel (Poland), Carolyn Shelton (South Africa), Deepika

Eranjanie Attygalle (Sri Lanka), Sutayut Osornprasop (Thailand), and Ahmet Levent Yener (Turkey). Some of these cases are being published as GDI case studies.

The team is grateful for background research by the following consultants: Vanessa Oddo, Manuela Villar Uribe, Ana Perez Esposito, Charlotte Block, and Claudia Trezza. The report was peer reviewed by Arturo Ardila Gomez (Global Lead, Urban Mobility, Transport GP); Asa Giertz (Senior Economist, Agriculture GP); Son Nam Nguyen (Lead Health Specialist, Health, Nutrition and Population GP); Veronica Silva (Senior Economist, Social Protection and Jobs GP); and Owen Smith (Senior Economist, Health, Nutrition and Population GP). The decision review meeting was chaired by Fadia Saadah (Director, Human Development) and Roberta Gatti (Chief Economist, Human Development).

The team thanks Hope Steele for her incredibly skilled editing, done at rapid speed, and her patience with the technical terms and abbreviations. Thanks to Nicole Hamam for preparing the graphics.

Financial support for this work was provided by the government of Japan through the Japan Trust Fund for Scaling Up Nutrition.

About the Editors

Barry Popkin is the W. R. Kenan, Jr. Distinguished Professor of Nutrition at the University of North Carolina at Chapel Hill (UNC). He developed the concept of the Nutrition Transition—the study of the dynamic shifts in our environment and the way they affect dietary intake, physical activity patterns and trends, and obesity and other nutrition-related non-communicable diseases. His research program focuses globally on understanding the shifts in stages of the transition and programs and policies to improve the population health linked with this transition (see www.nutrans.org). He is actively involved in work on the program and policy design and evaluation in the United States and globally, including collaborative research with colleagues in Brazil, Chile, Colombia, Mexico, and South Africa, for example (see Global Food Research Program at http://globalfoodresearchprogram.web .unc.edu/). He has a PhD in economics. He has received many major awards for his global contributions, including the 2016 World Obesity Society: Population Science and Public Health Award for top global public health researcher, the UK Rank Science Prize, and the Friends of Mickey Stunkard Lifetime Achievement Award of the Obesity Society.

Meera Shekar is Global Lead for nutrition with the World Bank's Health, Nutrition and Population Global Practice, managing key partnerships and firmly positioning nutrition within the World Bank's new initiative on Human Capital. She steered the repositioning of the nutrition agenda that led to the new global Scaling Up Nutrition (SUN) movement (https:// scalingupnutrition.org) and was a founding member of the Catalytic Financing Facility for Nutrition that evolved into the Power of Nutrition (https://www.powerofnutrition.org). She is chair of the SUN executive committee and has been one of the principals for the aid-architecture for nutrition within the G-8 and G-20 agenda-setting process. She led the development of the first global Investment Framework for Nutrition (https://open knowledge.worldbank.org/handle/10986/26069) and co-leads (with the Bill and Melinda Gates Foundation) the Nutrition Financing working group for the Nutrition for Growth (N4G) summit (https://nutritionforgrowth .org) to be hosted by Japan in 2020. She has a PhD in international nutrition, epidemiology, and population studies from Cornell University; has consulted and published extensively; and is on various advisory boards and panels, including the Essential Living Standards index (forthcoming; Legatum Institute, UK; and the advisory group at Gates Ventures.

Abbreviations

ANSA	Strategy against Overweight and Obesity (of Mexico)
BMI	body mass index
EAT	EAT Foundation
FAO	Food and Agriculture Organization of the United Nations
GDP	gross domestic product
GST	goods and services tax
NCDs	non-communicable diseases
NCD-RisC	NCD Risk Factor Collaboration
NGO	nongovernmental organization
PAHO	Pan-American Health Organization
SSBs	sugar-sweetened beverages
UNICEF	United Nations Children's Fund
VAT	value added tax
WHO	World Health Organization

Glossary

adult survival rate (ASR)
The *adult survival rate* (ASR) is one of the four indicators included in the Human Capital Index (HCI) developed by the World Bank (see page 24 for more details of the HCI). ASR is defined as the fraction of 15-year-olds that survive to age 60 and is used as a proxy for the range of non-fatal health outcomes that a child born today would experience as an adult if current conditions prevail into the future.[1]

body mass index (BMI)
Body mass index (BMI) is an index of weight-for-height commonly used to classify overweight and obesity on a large population basis, measured in a person's weight in kilograms divided by the square of his/her height in meters (kg/m^2). In adults, overweight is defined as a BMI of 25 or more, whereas obesity is a BMI of 30 or more.

diet-related tax
Diet-related taxes are implemented as a way to use fiscal policies, particularly taxation, to alter retail prices in such a way that sales and consumption of foods associated with diet-related non-communicable diseases are optimized. For example, taxes are levied on foods high in specific nutrients/ingredients (salt/fats/sugar) or otherwise classified as "unhealthy," including sugar-sweetened beverages. It could also take the form of reduced taxes (or subsidies) to promote the increased consumption of healthier food items, such as fruits and vegetables.

disability-adjusted life years (DALYs)
Disability-adjusted life years (DALYs) are a metric developed to quantify the overall disease burden from mortality and morbidity. DALYs for a particular disease or health condition are calculated as the sum of the years of life lost (YLL) due to premature mortality in the population and the years lost due to disability (YLD) for people living with the health condition or its consequences. One DALY can be thought of as one lost year of "healthy" life. DALYs of a population serve as a measurement of the gap between current health status and an ideal health situation—that is, disease burden—and allows us to estimate such gaps at the country, regional, and global levels.

double burden of malnutrition (DBM)	The *double burden of malnutrition* (DBM) is characterized by the coexistence of more than one serious nutritional problem within individuals, households, and/or populations, and across the life course. It is often referred to as *coexistence of undernutrition along with overweight and obesity*, or *diet-related non-communicable diseases,* while it could also include other forms of malnutrition, such as anemia and wasting. The term *triple burden of malnutrition* is also used when a population group simultaneously suffers from high levels of undernutrition, overweight/obesity, and micronutrient deficiencies such as anemia.

Global Nutrition Targets	In 2012, World Health Assembly Resolution 65.6 endorsed a comprehensive implementation plan on maternal, infant, and young child nutrition, which specified a set of six nutrition targets, known as *Global Nutrition Targets*, to be attained by 2025. The six targets are

1. Achieve a 40 percent reduction in the number of children under five who are stunted
2. Achieve a 50 percent reduction of anemia in women of reproductive age
3. Achieve a 30 percent reduction in low birth weight
4. Ensure that there is no increase in childhood overweight
5. Increase the rate of exclusive breastfeeding in the first six months up to at least 50 percent
6. Reduce and maintain childhood wasting to less than 5 percent

non-communicable diseases (NCDs)	*Non-communicable diseases* (NCDs) in a broader sense means diseases of non-transmissible/infectious nature, yet they are more commonly referred to as *chronic diseases* that tend to be of long duration and are the result of a combination of genetic, physiological, environmental, and behavioral factors. The four main types of NCDs are cardiovascular disease, diabetes, cancer, and chronic lung disease; together they are collectively responsible for almost 70 percent of all deaths worldwide.
	We refer to NCDs related to diet and nutrition as *diet-related NCDs*, which include cardiovascular disease (such as heart attacks and stroke, and often linked to high blood pressure), diabetes, and certain cancers. Unhealthy diets and poor nutrition are among the top risk factors for these diseases globally.

nutrition transition	*Nutrition transition* in a population describes progressive shifts in the stages of eating, drinking, and moving from traditional, nutrient-rich diets to energy-dense, nutrient-poor, ultra-processed foods, sugary calorie-laden beverages, and increased sedentary lifestyle that coincides with or is preceded by economic, demographic, and epidemiological changes. Sociodemographic characteristics, such as income, education, sex, and location, can often predict which segments of the population will be worst affected by the nutrition transition, but this will depend on the macro- and microeconomic forces and sociocultural aspects inherent to each region.

overweight and obesity	*Overweight and obesity* result from an imbalance between energy consumed (too much) and energy expended (too little). Globally, people are consuming foods and drinks that are more energy dense (high in sugars and fats) and engaging in less physical activity.

To define the state of overweight and/or obesity for adults ages 18 years and older, there are age- and gender-specific cutoffs delineated by the WHO, the U.S. Centers for Disease Control and Prevention (CDC), and the International Obesity Task Force (IOTF) that are used in different studies, countries, and contexts. The prevalence differences overall in these methods are small. Using the WHO's cutoffs, overweight and/or obesity are commonly defined by the following:

- Overweight: BMI $\geq$ 25 kg/m^2, < 30 kg/m^2
- Obesity: BMI $\geq$ 30 kg/m^2
- Overweight and obesity (overweight/obesity): BMI $\geq$ 25 kg/m^2

For children, particularly in preschool ages, overweight/obesity is defined as 2 standard deviations from the median of the WHO Child Growth Standards measured in weight-for-length/height z-scores (this definition is universally used in this report).

sin tax

A *sin tax* is an excise or ad valorem tax specifically levied on certain goods deemed harmful to society and individuals—for example, alcohol, tobacco, sugar-sweetened/soda drinks, fast foods, and gambling, among others—to increase their price in an effort to lower their use and reduce the negative impacts of the taxed substance.

sugar-
sweetened
beverages
(SSB)

Sugar-sweetened beverages (SSBs) are any liquids that are sweetened with added sugars (for example, brown sugar, corn sweetener, corn syrup, dextrose, fructose, glucose, high-fructose corn syrup, honey, lactose, malt syrup, maltose, molasses, raw sugar, and sucrose), such as regular non-sugar-free soda, fruit/sports/energy drinks, sweetened waters, and coffee/tea beverages with added sugars. The calories in SSBs can contribute to weight gain and provide little to no nutritional value and lead to other health risks including obesity, tooth decay, heart disease, and type 2 diabetes. SSBs are associated with minimal effect on hunger, so consuming sugary drinks is not expected to reduce food intake. With an aim of reducing the consumption of SSBs, the sales of the defined products are regulated—for example, they are restricted on school premises or taxed as an important public health measure.

stunting

Stunting is a chronic form of undernutrition (as opposed to an acute form of undernutrition, called *wasting*), which often occurs as a result of the accumulation/recurrence of damaging conditions such as poor socioeconomic status, poor maternal health and nutrition, frequent illness, and/or inappropriate infant and young child feeding and care in early life. Stunting is known to affect children's physical and cognitive development and consequently their health and productivity in their adulthood.

A child is categorized as *stunted* when her/his length or height-for-age z-score is below –2 standard deviations based on the WHO Child Growth Standards. Child stunting is also used in the Human Capital Index as an indicator for the prenatal, infant, and early childhood health environment, summarizing the risks to good health that children born today are likely to experience in their early years—with important consequences for health and well-being in adulthood.

syndemic   A *syndemic* or synergistic epidemic is the aggregation of two or more concurrent or sequential epidemics or disease clusters in a population with biological interactions, which exacerbate the prognosis and burden of disease, in this case referring to the global syndemic of undernutrition, overweight/obesity, and climate change.

Note

1. Aart Kraay. 2018. "Methodology for a World Bank Human Capital Index." Policy Research Working Paper 8593, World Bank, Washington, DC. http://documents.worldbank.org/curated/en/300071537907028892/pdf/WPS8593.pdf.

Executive Summary

What This Report Does

This report lays out why overweight and obesity is a "ticking time bomb" with huge potential negative economic and health impacts, especially for the poor and people who live in low- or middle-income countries, dispelling the myth that it is a problem only in high-income countries and urban areas. The report also lays out many of the current trends concerning overweight and obesity and complements all of the new and forthcoming technical reports on this issue in four distinct ways:

- First, it focuses on identifying evidence-based opportunities for fiscal and regulatory policy reforms and investments across several sectors that could potentially prevent overweight and obesity. In doing so, it builds on the epidemiological evidence from several technical reports to identify potentially promising actions; adds new information on the economic implications of overweight and obesity, including the equity perspective, that may be useful in making the case for action; and identifies the growing list of "double-burden" countries to spur urgent action in these countries.
- Second, it brings to bear implementation challenges and lessons learned from several country case studies where policies or interventions to prevent overweight and obesity have been rolled out at scale, with variable success.
- Third, and perhaps most important, it identifies an action agenda—specifically on the unique role that client countries, with support from institutions such as the World Bank, can play in this space—and the

1

instruments (policy and regulatory levers, technical assistance, and results-based financing instruments as well as investment lending) that the World Bank (and other similar institutions) can use in the near future to support countries in addressing the emerging epidemic of overweight and obesity and related non-communicable diseases (NCDs) across sectors.

- Fourth, the report reiterates research findings from recent technical reports from the *Lancet* that suggest that changing diets and food systems are also key to addressing the ongoing challenge of child stunting and undernutrition, along with the growing challenges of climate change. It also identifies key areas requiring further research and evaluations that may be important for future actions in this area.

Obesity: The Problem Defined

Overweight and obesity result from an imbalance between energy consumed (too much) and energy expended (too little). Globally, there has been a shift in food consumption patterns whereby people are consuming more energy-dense foods (those high in sugars and fats); at the same time, they are engaging in significantly reduced physical activity. Using the World Health Organization's (WHO's) cutoffs, adults with a body mass index (BMI; this is weight/height squared) of 25 or more are classified as overweight; those with a BMI of 30 or more are classified as obese. The terms *overweight* and *obesity* both identify people who are at risk for health problems from having too much body fat (see also the glossary). For simplicity, this executive summary uses the term *obesity* to refer to both conditions.

The ticking time bomb of obesity has huge potential economic and health impacts, especially for the poor. As of 2016, an estimated 44 percent of adults (more than 2 billion) worldwide are overweight or obese, and over 70 percent of them live in low- or middle-income countries (see map ES.1 and figure ES.1).

Over 70 percent of countries—the vast majority of which are low- and lower-middle-income countries—currently face a double burden: a high prevalence of both undernutrition and obesity. As per capita income increases, the burden of obesity shifts to the poor and to rural areas across low- and middle-income countries. Over 55 percent of the global rise in obesity is found in rural areas; in South East Asia, Latin America, Central Asia, and North Africa this increase is close to 80 or 90 percent of the recent shift. This has significantly closed the urban-rural gap in most regions except Sub-Saharan Africa. Today most of the countries in the world with high levels of the double burden are found in Sub-Saharan Africa, South Asia, selected South East Asian countries (Indonesia being most prominent), and Guatemala. This is a marked shift from the 1990s, when Mexico and most of Central America, Bolivia, Peru, South Africa, Francophone Africa, the Arab Republic of Egypt, parts of Central Asia, and the Philippines faced severe levels of the double burden.

In addition, in many low- and middle-income countries, for an array of genetic and epi-genetic reasons, populations are more susceptible to NCDs at BMI levels lower than 25 (overweight).

Map ES.1   Overweight/Obesity Prevalence by Country Income Level

a. Low- and Middle-Income Countries

1990s

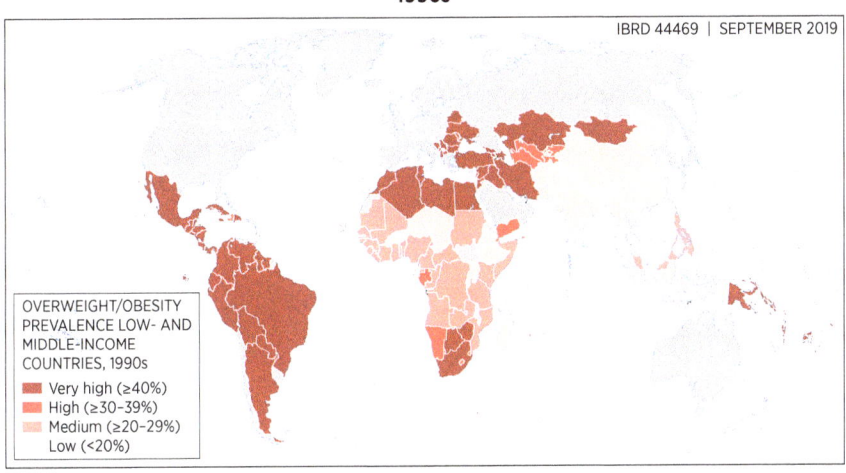

2010s

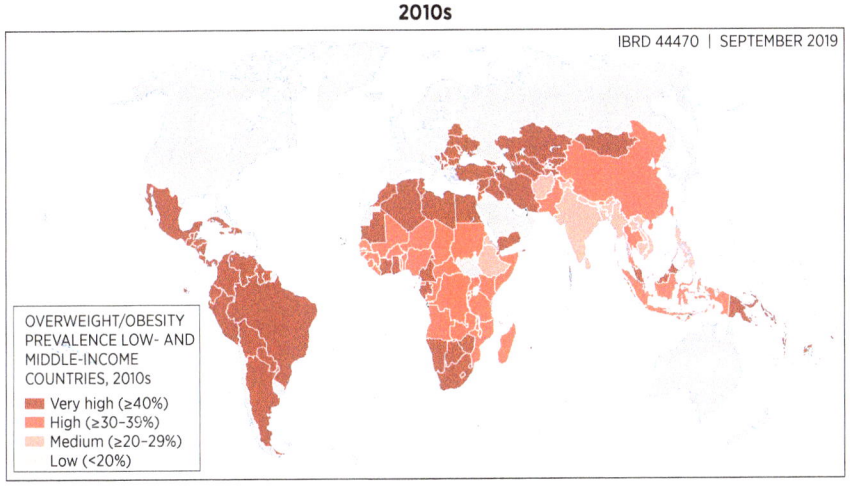

continued next page

Map ES.1 *(continued)*

b. High-Income Countries
1990s

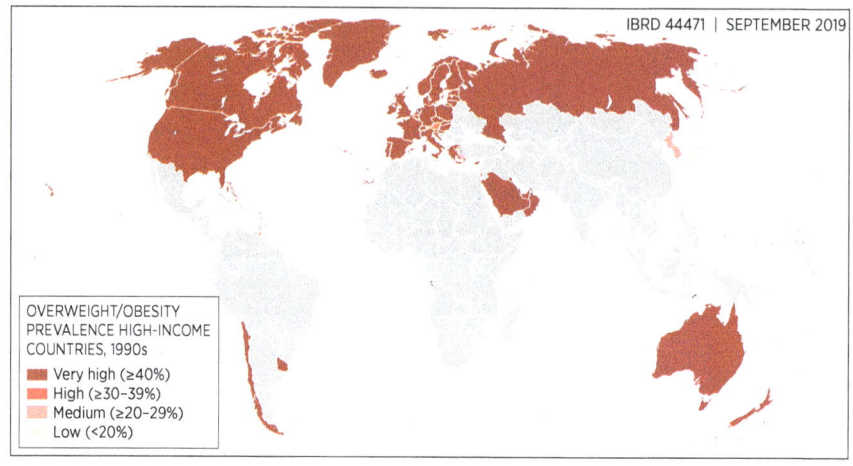

2010s

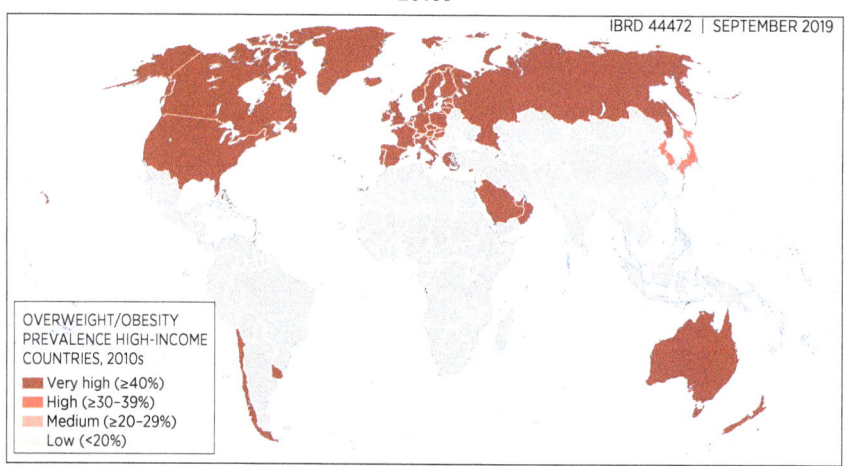

Sources: Popkin, Global Food Research Program, University of North Carolina. Data are from UNICEF, WHO, World Bank, and NCD-RisC estimates, supplemented with selected Demographic and Health Surveys and other country direct national measures.

Note: Based on 1990s and 2010s weight and height data.

Childhood obesity is particularly damaging. It puts the child at high risk of developing debilitating NCDs earlier in life and living with them longer, denying the child her or his full health and economic potential. It also puts in place a trajectory of poor diet and activity patterns that accentuate the risks of increased weight gain. Concurrently, stunting and poor growth

Figure ES.1   More Than Three-Quarters of Overweight or Obese Individuals Live in Middle-Income Countries

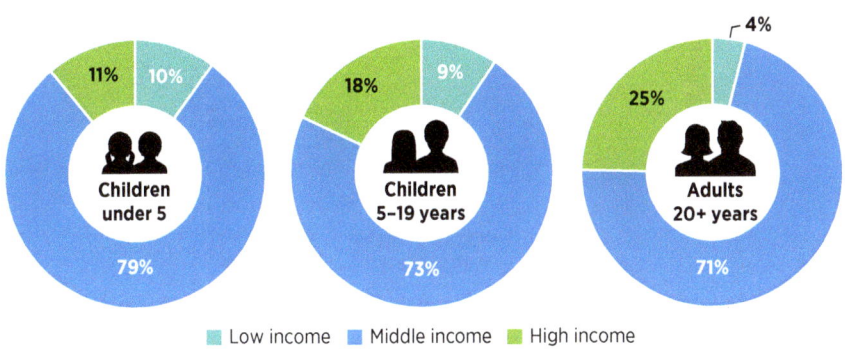

Sources: Data on overweight and obesity levels from NCD-RisC estimates for 2016, http://ncdrisc.org/data-downloads.html; country income classifications based on World Bank criteria as of 2015.

during the first 1,000 days of life significantly increase children's risks of accumulating visceral fat (obesity in central areas of the body) and many related NCDs later in life when they are exposed to a lifestyle dominated by ultra-processed foods and reduced physical activity. Consequently, many low-income countries are starting to suffer from the double burden of malnutrition—increases in overweight and obesity even as the burden of undernutrition remains high. The long-term costs of obesity and NCDs will be significantly exacerbated by the lag in the impact of current and past stunting reduction programs.

The Health and Economic Costs of Obesity

Increasing health care costs linked to increasing obesity rates are a trend across the world, and both overweight and obesity are significant risk factors for NCDs (see figure ES.2).

The critical issue in understanding the economic impacts of obesity is that mortality, albeit significantly increased, is not the only major outcome. Reduced productivity, increased disabilities, increased health care costs, early retirement, and reduced length of disability-free healthy living across the life cycle—all of which will impact human capital outcomes in countries—are also significant consequences. As obesity rates are rapidly increasing, global attention to this issue is increasing. Poor diets, a lack of physical activity, and overweight and obesity are now recognized as the top preventable causes of NCDs in all countries in the world.

The estimated economic costs of obesity vary considerably, since studies use different methodologies to estimate direct and indirect costs.

Figure ES.2 Health Impacts of Overweight/Obesity

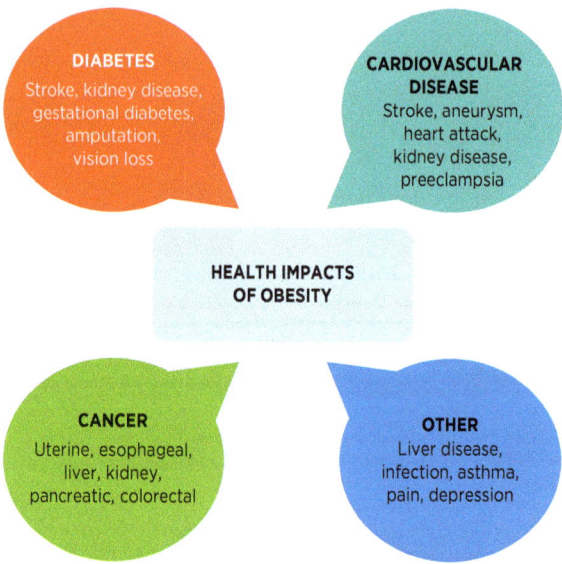

For example, estimates from the United States range from US$89 billion to US$212 billion in total costs; those from China are estimated at 3.58 and 8.73 percent of gross national product (GNP) in 2020 and 2025, respectively; and Brazil projects a doubling of the obesity-related health care costs from US$5.8 billion in 2010 to US$10.1 billion in 2050. The effects of obesity on productivity, early retirement, and disabilities have rarely been studied in low- and middle-income countries. In addition, the same poor diets dominated increasingly by ultra-processed foods and the reduced activity patterns that affect obesity increase the risk of a wide array of NCDs directly as well as indirectly.

Whatever estimates one might subscribe to, the big picture message is that increasing health care costs linked to increasing obesity rates are a trend across both the developed and the developing world. Preventing obesity therefore makes sense from a public finance perspective. Governments and development partners have a key role to play in this effort, including by ensuring that consumers are informed about the health and other consequences of their dietary and lifestyle choices.

Factors Affecting Obesity

Three sets of factors can affect overweight/obesity: (1) early life undernutrition and reduced linear growth, (2) reduced energy expenditure through changes in technology and lifestyles in all phases of life, and (3) a set of factors linked to changing food systems and the resultant shifts in food consumption and eating behaviors.

The analyses presented in this report suggest that a range of conditions that emerge with globalization, urbanization, and technological development are driving the rise in obesity rates globally:

- Rapid reductions in physical activity in all domains of activity, from market-related work and home production (for example, water gathering, food preparation/cooking) to transportation and leisure in low- and middle-income countries in the last 15–35 years, and global access to labor-reducing technologies.
- Rapid shifts in the built environment, which contributed both to reduced physical activity in many cases and to changes in the food environment.
- The spread of modern food retailing and a rapidly changing food system. This has led to major shifts toward diets dominated by ultra-processed foods, and was linked to higher price increases for healthy foods than for unhealthy products.
- Women entering the formal market labor force in large proportions in most high-income countries and in low- and middle-income countries, requiring changes in food consumption.
- Shifts in eating patterns, which have led to increased snacking and away-from-home eating.
- Increased country and household income, which have been linked to a shift to greater obesity among the poor in all high-income countries and in an increasing proportion of low- and middle-income countries.
- Increased wealth in many low-income countries, which has shifted them to middle-income countries and in some cases to high-income countries.
- Modern media and marketing that, along with globalization, has shifted social and cultural norms related to dietary and activity patterns.

Based on these emerging conditions, the conceptual framework below highlights the actionable direct and indirect factors associated with obesity (figure ES.3).

Opportunities to Address Obesity

The evidence base for preventing obesity is still emerging. Table ES.1 summarizes the promising interventions/policies that have the potential to prevent obesity. These include a range of:

1. fiscal policies such as taxation and subsidies;
2. regulatory policies on marketing and advertising (including direct marketing to children in schools);

Figure ES.3 Factors Affecting Overweight/Obesity: A Conceptual Framework

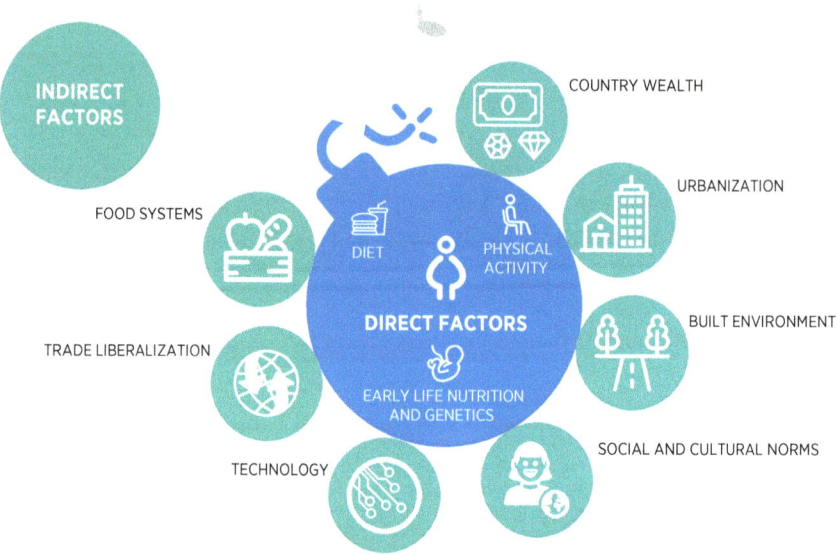

3. food systems approaches, including the proliferation of modern food retailing and away-from-home food service options—some formal and many informal;
4. education sector policies that affect areas such as school cafeterias, marketing, and sales of unhealthy food in and around schools, as well as physical activity in schools;
5. transport and urban design interventions such as mass transit and city and building design; and
6. early childhood nutrition programs to address undernutrition.

Unlike many other public-health interventions, very few of these policies or interventions (except for early childhood programs) have been rigorously evaluated, and they have not been and cannot be tested through randomized controlled trials. Few have undergone systematic reviews because their effectiveness has not yet been demonstrated or carefully documented. Nonetheless, initial assessments, a limited number of systematic reviews, and lessons from several countries suggest that the following policies/interventions are promising—not just for their potential impacts on preventing obesity, but also for potential climate co-benefits. In addition, there are a series of interventions that have been shown to impact undernutrition, such as breastfeeding promotion, that are also triple-duty actions in terms of their simultaneous impact on undernutrition, obesity, and climate change.

Table ES.1 Key Interventions with Potential for Impact

Policy Intervention type	Goal	Effectiveness demonstrated	Potential impact and scope of impact on target population
Fiscal policies			
Taxes/subsidies	Reduce consumption of ultra-processed foods and beverages, primary focus to date on sugar-sweetened beverage reduction	Chile, Mexico, United Kingdom, and South Africa [papers forthcoming]; U.S. cities	• Impact depends on the size/design of the tax • Nutrient-based taxes such as tiered taxes and taxes based on number of grams of sugar promote reformulation • Impactful in reducing consumption among high-volume consumers, with potential for prevention of overweight/obesity among children/adolescents
Regulatory policies on marketing and advertising			
Front-of-package warning labels	Reduce consumption of ultra-processed foods and beverages; change eating norms	Chile [unpublished series of papers forthcoming]	• Very impactful when combined with other linked policies • Universal targeting
Marketing controls on foods for children	Reduce consumption of ultra-processed foods and beverages; change eating norms	Chile, many others	• Potential for impact when linked to other policies • Can reduce child exposure; total family exposure does not change
Regulations on total marketing and sales of unhealthy foods	Reduce consumption of ultra-processed foods and beverages; change eating norms	Chile	• Potential for changing norms • Reaches all children; more impactful on younger children
Retailer interventions	Reduce consumption of ultra-processed foods and beverages	United States, United Kingdom	• Potential for high impact • Potential for important food purchase changes
Agriculture/food systems approaches			
Agriculture research	Incentivize research on underserved foods (legumes, fruits, vegetables)	CGIAR	• Potential for high impact • Potential to shift relative prices

continued next page

Table ES.1 (*continued*)

Policy Intervention type	Goal	Effectiveness demonstrated	Potential impact and scope of impact on target population
	Ensure agriculture research has a nutrition focus, not just a yield focus	CGIAR, country programs	• Potential high in general; only initial stages of efforts globally • Potential huge for shifting relative food prices
Agriculture subsidies	Eliminate subsidies for unhealthy ingredients (for example, sugar, corn, palm oil)	Yet to be implemented	• Potential impact unclear for shifting relative prices; but could provide fiscal benefits for countries
Food processing	Build awareness of unhealthy ingredients used in food processing	Yet to be implemented	• Potential impact unclear
Formal food service sector	Reduce consumption of ultra-processed foods and beverages	None	• Potentially impactful • As income increases, the proportion of meals eaten outside the home increases rapidly, so the potential impact rises • Dependent on laws impacting pricing policies, labeling, sizing
Informal food service sector	Reduce consumption of ultra-processed foods and beverages	Singapore	• Great potential but requires experimentation (existing experience shows limited impact as focus is on sanitation, healthy oils; no pricing/portion controls used)
Education sector approaches			
School food service quality and school premises sales regulations	Reduce consumption of ultra-processed foods and beverages; change eating norms for children	CGIAR, country programs	• Potential high; only initial stages of efforts globally • Potential huge for shifting relative food prices
Active transport and building/city design			
Mass transit system	Increase movement, energy expenditure	None	• Minimal potential for impact on overweight/obesity but important for health and climate • Mostly affects low- and middle-income populations

continued next page

Table ES.1 (*continued*)

Policy Intervention type	Goal	Effectiveness demonstrated	Potential impact and scope of impact on target population
City design: parks, cycling lanes	Increase movement, energy expenditure	Colombia, Netherlands, United Kingdom	• Potential for impact among users
Building design to enhance walking	Increase movement, energy expenditure	Europe, United States, Australia	• Minimal impact on overweight/obesity but important for health • Potential for increasing physical activity
Early childhood nutrition programs			
Breastfeeding promotion	Improve breastfeeding rates	Many countries	• Impact global as documented across many low-, middle-, and high-income countries
Prevention of early childhood stunting	Well-documented package of interventions across sectors	Many countries	• Relevant mostly for low-income countries and some middle-income countries

Note: CGIAR = Consultative Group on International Agricultural Research.

Country Experience to Date

While fiscal policies linked mainly to taxation on sugar-sweetened beverages have dominated as key interventions in over 40 countries to reduce consumption of unhealthy foods (see map ES.2) and there is extensive experience in this area, many other regulatory options are being used by countries to improve diet quality (map ES.3). These include front-of-package labeling, nutrient profiling, school-based food regulations and education, market and retail solutions, and marketing controls and regulations.

Front-of-package labeling and related nutrition profiling models with warning labels show great promise; diet-related taxes also remain a promising approach, albeit they will face challenges. The main challenges to the successful implementation of these taxes are a tax system's administrative capacity, substitution effects, tax evasion, and opposition from the food industry. These challenges need to be considered when designing effective tax policies. Countries with strong tax administration generally design excise taxes based on nutrient content, albeit taxes on product volumes may be easier to implement in countries where tax administration is not so strong. Tiered tax systems based on sugar content appear to be another promising approach. And experience suggests

Map ES.2 Sugar-Sweetened Beverage Taxes around the World

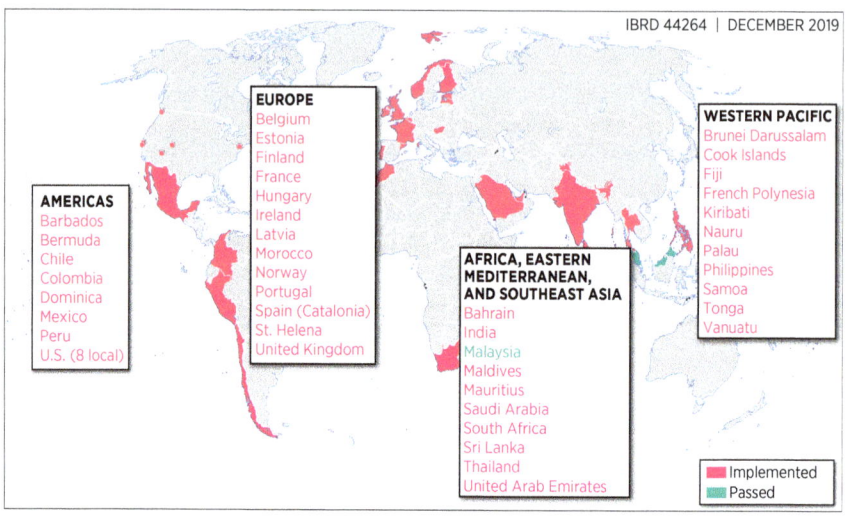

Source: Global Food Research Program, University of North Carolina, http://globalfood researchprogram.web.unc.edu/multi-country-initiative/resources/.

Note: This map was created based on the dataset available as of March 2019.

that a regional approach to taxation will likely reduce cross-border purchases and prevent resulting tax evasion. A combination of policies, such as those in Chile, promise important synergies and much larger impacts.

No countries have yet considered tying the taxes to subsidies for healthier legumes, vegetables, and fruits and other healthful, less obesogenic foods, although earmarking sin taxes for public programs brings even more challenges. Experience in marketing regulation of unhealthy foods is also limited, except perhaps what has been learned from the marketing of infant formulas. However, new research emerging from Chile will shed more light on this approach, suggesting that carefully designed laws may be impactful on exposure to obesogenic foods. Furthermore, emerging evidence also suggests that impacts of such obesity-prevention policies are starting to be realized. For example, the 10 percent tax on sugar-sweetened beverages in Mexico is estimated to reduce obesity by 2.5 percent by 2024 and prevent 86,000 to 134,000 new cases of diabetes by 2030; another study estimated a reduction of 189,300 fewer cases of type 2 diabetes, 20,400 fewer cases of strokes and myocardial infarctions, and 18,900 fewer deaths occurring from 2013 to 2022 in Mexico as a result of this taxation.

Map ES.3 Countries with Mandatory or Voluntary Front-of-Package Labels

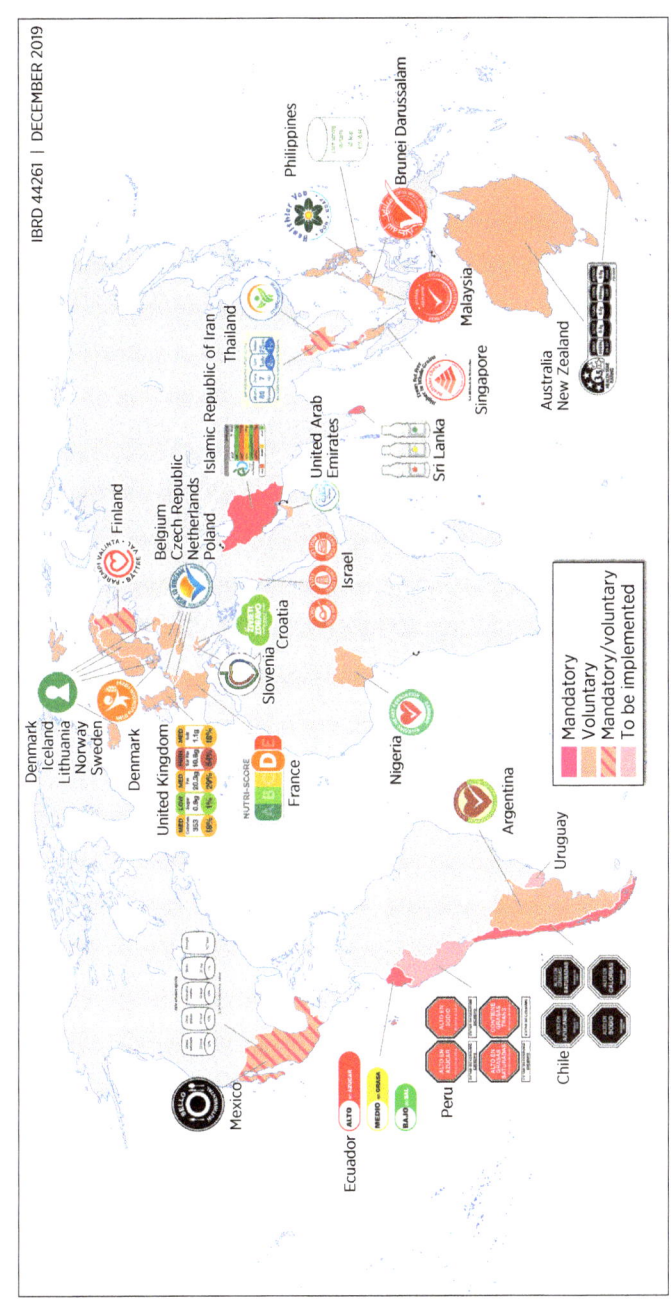

IBRD 44261 | DECEMBER 2019

Source: Global Food Research Program, University of North Carolina, 2019, http://globalfoodresearchprogram.web.unc.edu/multi-country-initiative/resources/.

Note: This map was created based on the dataset available as of March 2019.

Important shifts in urban planning and design are also being undertaken. All forms of design that increase physical activity—from building design that makes stairs an attractive option to urban design that incentivizes and enables biking and walking—are important. Reducing car use and increasing mass transit/biking/walking are major global needs, which also have significant climate co-benefits. However, current experience with improved physical activity and obesity prevention is limited to a handful of countries, mostly in the global north and South America. While these are promising strategies, future efforts need to build in evaluation of large-scale urban or national programs to document their impacts. There are no evaluations as yet equivalent to the Mexican or Chilean rigorous evaluations of their food-related fiscal and regulatory policies in the physical activity domain.

It is also important to note that this is the beginning of large-scale policies and regulations designed by countries to improve diet quality, increase physical activity, and prevent obesity, and so to contribute to healthy living throughout the life cycle. Many of these policies and regulations will have significant climate co-benefits as well. In the first half of the 2010s, over 50 countries have engaged in some major fiscal policy or regulatory action in this area. Many evaluations currently underway will assist in providing evidence on which approaches may also have the greatest impact on water use and carbon emissions, but major gaps still exist between the evidence concerning impact and best practices today.

Conclusions and Next Steps

The global obesity epidemic presents a formidable challenge to human capital acquisition, national wealth accumulation, and the goals of ending extreme poverty and boosting shared prosperity. While reductions in undernutrition are being observed globally and investments in reducing undernutrition are at an all-time high, obesity rates are rising rapidly.

Continued economic growth among the world's low- and middle-income countries will only intensify the magnitude of the devastating impacts of obesity on health, well-being, and productivity. Furthermore, as economies grow, the burden of obesity will shift even more toward the poor, making it all the more imperative for the global development community, including institutions such as the World Bank, to engage.

Obesity has a large impact on national economies—both through reduced productivity, increased disability, and reduced life expectancy, and through significantly increased health care costs. The effort to reduce obesity is therefore a global public good and governments have a key role to play in addressing this challenge through a comprehensive approach to policy formulation and intervention, including in the agriculture, environment, transport, education, fiscal, and health care sectors.

Recent technical reports from the *Lancet* suggest that, in addition to addressing obesity, changing diets and food systems are also key to addressing the growing challenges of climate change as well as the ongoing challenge of child stunting and undernutrition. The shift in diets and activity patterns globally linked to increased obesity are also linked to important water and carbon emissions concerns, thus perpetuating what is termed by the *Lancet* Commission on Obesity as the *syndemic of undernutrition, overweight/obesity, and climate change*.

The good news is that there are also potential double- and triple-duty actions that will provide climate co-benefits in addition to being promising interventions to address obesity and undernutrition. For example, sugar is one of the more water-intensive crops, and reduced sugar consumption is expected to lead to important reductions in water use and related climate co-benefits. The *Lancet* EAT Commission report also advocates a shift toward more sustainable plant-based diets to address both obesity and climate change. The World Bank has the ability to work across these sectors and to help guide countries toward fiscal and regulatory policies as well as investment policies to prevent further increases in obesity, while also tackling undernutrition and climate change through double-duty and triple-duty actions that have an impact on undernutrition, obesity, and climate change.

Countries need to act urgently to address obesity. Development partners such as the World Bank are in a unique position to support low-, middle-, and high-income client countries to better prevent obesity. In their engagement with country governments, development partners can highlight the issue of obesity as one requiring corrective public action rather than one of individual responsibility. And agencies such as the World Bank can transform this advocacy into tangible investment opportunities through the repertoire of analytical, diagnostic, policy, technical assistance, and investment tools that can be deployed to address different aspects of the obesity challenges.

Given the renewed global focus on human capital, its links to the obesity epidemic, and the growing evidence base for double- and triple-duty actions, there are both an urgent need and great opportunities for advocacy and action at scale. The health sector needs to lead on diagnostics, but tackling this complex agenda will require both a whole-of-government and a whole-of-development-partner approach, with the agriculture, transport, macroeconomics, trade and investment, and education sectors each having a major role to play.

Figure ES.4 Strategic Areas for Potential Development Partners Action

STRATEGIC AREA 1
Leveraging the range of tools at global/regional/country levels

STRATEGIC AREA 2
Scaling up promising interventions and policies, and supporting reforms through multisectoral engagement, including through the private sector

STRATEGIC AREA 3
Building the evidence and knowledge base across sectors

OBESITY PREVENTION

STRATEGIC AREAS

FOR POTENTIAL INVOLVEMENT OF DEVELOPMENT PARTNERS TO SUPPORT COUNTRIES

The report concludes that client countries, with support from development partners such as the World Bank, are well positioned to address the economic and health consequences of obesity. There are three key strategic areas in which these agencies, including the World Bank, can support countries to maximize their impact (figure ES.4):

- Strategic Area 1: Leveraging the range of advocacy, policy, and investment tools available to countries and development partners at global, regional, and country levels
- Strategic Area 2: Scaling up promising interventions and policies, and supporting reforms through multisectoral engagement, including through the private sector
- Strategic Area 3: Building the evidence and knowledge base across sectors to document impacts and best practices on how to implement these policies/interventions

The following five key areas are identified as critical for further research and analysis by countries and development partners:

- Documenting the impact of fiscal and regulatory policies and cross-sectoral interventions in countries where these are being applied, including a focus on how these can be adapted in different country contexts
- Quantifying the climate co-benefits of investing in obesity prevention policies and programs
- Building the evidence base for food systems approaches to prevent obesity
- Instigating stronger engagement with the private sector
- Quantifying the contribution of obesity to adult survival rates and the Human Capital Index

Small tweaks to current engagement models will not be sufficient. A transformative approach and additional financial and human resources need to be dedicated to this agenda by all countries, as well as by development partners. Building internal capacity within client countries as well as within partners such as the World Bank to work across sectoral boundaries and with nontraditional partners will be crucial. The experience with tobacco suggests that this will be a long road, but it is feasible, in consultation with like-minded global and national partners such as Bloomberg Philanthropies, the EAT Foundation, UN partners such as the WHO and UNICEF, and academia and civil society.

1

Why This Report Now?

Meera Shekar

Key Messages

- Global attention to overweight/obesity has recently burgeoned. Increases in the incidence of overweight/obesity are accelerating in most low- and middle-income countries. The impact of overweight/obesity on productivity and economic development is huge in terms of increased health care costs, reduced productivity, disability, early retirement, and life expectancy. Unhealthy diets, physical inactivity, and overweight/obesity jointly represent the top preventable causes of non-communicable diseases (NCDs) in all countries in the world.
- Recent technical reports from two *Lancet* commissions suggest that changing diets and food systems are also key to addressing the growing challenges of climate change as well as the ongoing challenge of child stunting and undernutrition.
- Governments have a key role to play in addressing these challenges by providing a comprehensive approach to policy formulation and intervention, including in the agriculture, environment, transport, taxation, and health care sectors.
- Development partners such as the World Bank, foundations, and UN agencies have the ability to help guide countries toward fiscal, regulatory, and investment policies to prevent further increases in overweight/obesity while also tackling undernutrition and climate change—a trilogy of effects referred to as a *syndemic* by the 2019 *Lancet* Commission on Obesity (LCO).

- This report builds on the many new and forthcoming technical reports on overweight/obesity prevention to identify an action agenda for institutions such as the World Bank that are uniquely positioned to act across sectoral boundaries (including the health, agriculture, macro/fiscal, urban design/city planning, and education sectors, among others) and to deploy both policy and investment tools to address this wake-up call.

Overweight/Obesity: A Ticking Time Bomb

Overweight/obesity is a time bomb ready to explode. Overweight/obesity rates are high and increasing rapidly across the world, in both developed and developing economies, and the burden is growing rapidly in every region of the world. Worldwide, as of 2016, an estimated 44 percent of adults (more than 2 billion) are overweight/obese; over 70 percent of them live in low- or middle-income countries, dispelling the myth that overweight/obesity is a problem in high-income countries alone. The burden of overweight/obesity has nearly tripled since 1975 and now accounts annually for about 4 million deaths globally (The GBD 2015 Obesity Collaborators 2017). And rural overweight/obesity is growing rapidly in many developing countries. Over the next several decades these trends are likely to increase significantly unless urgent actions are taken to curtail this progression. Furthermore, as countries grow economically and per capita incomes rise, the burden is shifting even more toward the poor, with potentially devastating impacts on the health of the poor, on the need for financial protection especially for the poor, and on overall economic development. In-depth and broader studies on overweight/obesity have shown how an increased shift of a higher burden of overweight/obesity among the poor has been linked with increased gross domestic product (GDP) per capita in low- and middle-income countries (Jones-Smith et al. 2011, 2012). In addition, in the new *Lancet* series on the double burden of malnutrition (DBM), the lead study shows how the bottom quartile in GDP per capita countries have been most likely to have the highest levels of DBM compared with other countries, while in the 1990s the top quartile countries were most likely to have high levels of DBM (Popkin, Corvalan, and Grummer-Strawn 2019). These are mainly countries in South Asia and Sub-Saharan Africa plus Indonesia. Whichever way it is examined, increasing health care costs linked to increasing overweight/obesity rates are a trend across the world.

A Drain on National Economies and an Imperative for Government Action

Estimates of the economic costs of overweight/obesity suggest a wide range because the methods used to estimate these costs vary considerably—some studies base their estimates on the direct medical costs of treatment while others include indirect costs linked to disability, increased mortality, and reduced productivity (often termed *presenteeism* in the literature; Trogdon et al. 2008). An unpublished systematic review of published studies conducted for this report identified 34 studies between 2007 and 2017 that estimated the national costs of overweight, obesity, or both. These studies cover 13 high- and middle-income countries. The results suggest a wide range of estimated costs in terms of share of GDP lost: from 0.01 percent in Brazil to 2.08 percent in the United States. Another estimate from the United States suggests that overweight/obesity costs the government, employers, and individuals about US$147 billion per year; further, this cost will rise significantly as medical treatment for chronic diseases becomes more sophisticated. An estimate from Indonesia (Kosen 2018) suggests losses of about 3 percent of GDP, equivalent to about US$28.4 billion; another global estimate suggests losses of 2.8 percent of GDP, equal to about US$2.0 trillion (Dobbs et al. 2014).

Whatever the final estimates, the costs are high, and—combined with the fact that overweight/obesity rates in the United States are growing and life expectancy is declining (especially compared with countries such as France, Germany, Japan, and the United Kingdom)—this should be a cause for major concern among policy makers. In Germany, the direct costs of overweight/obesity were estimated at €8,647 million in 2008, corresponding to 3.27 percent of total German heath care expenditures, with additional indirect costs of €8,150 million, of which two-thirds were costs of unpaid work linked to sickness-related absences, early retirement, and early mortality (Lehnert et al. 2015).

In China, estimates of increased health care costs associated with overweight/obesity have grown from 0.56 percent of China's annual national health care expenditure in 2000 to 3.13 percent in 2009 (Qin and Pan 2016). Another estimate in China that looked at the total costs of overweight/obesity found that the indirect costs of overweight/obesity and overweight/obesity-related dietary and physical activity patterns ranged from 3.58 percent of gross national product in 2000 to a projected 8.73 percent in 2025 (Popkin et al. 2006). In Brazil, overweight/obesity-related health care costs are expected to nearly double, from US$5.8 billion in 2010 to US$10.1 billion in 2050. Increasing health care costs linked to increasing overweight/obesity rates are a trend across the world. Investing in the prevention of overweight/obesity therefore makes sense from a public finance perspective—it would help save resources in the health sector and improve national productivity (Rtveladze et al. 2013).

Furthermore, many proposed interventions to reduce overweight/obesity will have important positive implications for reducing water use and greenhouse gas emissions, thereby also providing significant climate co-benefits. For example, sugar is one of the more water-intensive crops, and reduced sugar consumption is expected to lead to important reductions in water use (Constantino-Toto and Montero 2016; Ercin, Aldaya, and Hoekstra 2011). The EAT-*Lancet* Commission report (2019) suggests that dietary shifts to less meat consumption will not only reduce overweight/obesity rates but will also significantly reduce greenhouse gas production. The *Lancet* Commission report "Global Syndemic of Obesity, Undernutrition, and Climate Change" (LCO 2019) suggests a series of double- and triple-duty actions that have the potential to address overweight/obesity, undernutrition, and climate change simultaneously. None of the estimated economic benefits of overweight/obesity prevention as yet build in these huge potential climate co-benefits.

Preventing overweight/obesity is therefore a global public good from both public finance and health perspectives. Furthermore, governments have a key role to play: they can intervene to ensure consumers are informed about the health consequences of their dietary choices and can correct for large differences in relative prices. Equity issues and market failure present an additional argument for government intervention to prevent overweight/obesity. For example, although most sin taxes or taxes on ultra-processed food and beverages may be regressive in economic terms, they are progressive from a health perspective in that they prevent overweight/obesity and the related NCDs in the population with the highest burden of NCDs overall as well as the highest burden of untreated NCDs. Emerging evidence suggests that the impacts of such policies are starting to be realized. For example, the 10 percent tax on sugar-sweetened beverages in Mexico is estimated to reduce overweight/obesity by 2.5 percent by 2024 and to prevent 86,000 to 134,000 new cases of diabetes by 2030, while another study estimated 189,300 fewer cases of type 2 diabetes, 20,400 fewer cases of strokes and myocardial infarctions, and 18,900 fewer deaths occurring from 2013 to 2022 (Barrientos-Gutierrez et al. 2017; Sánchez-Romero et al. 2016).

Global Attention to Overweight/Obesity

In recent years, overweight/obesity has come to the fore on the global development agenda. The Sustainable Development Goals (SDGs) make reference to overweight and obesity under SDG target 2.2, which aims to end all forms of malnutrition (including overweight and obesity) by 2030.

The World Health Assembly in 2012 adopted six new nutrition targets, including "to ensure that there is no increase in childhood overweight by 2025" (WHO 2014a). The WHO has also issued several other recent reports, including the *Global Action Plan for the Prevention and Control of Noncommunicable Diseases 2013–2020* (WHO 2013) and the "Global Nutrition Targets 2025: Childhood Overweight" Policy Brief (WHO 2014b), among others, which provide a road map of policies and interventions to meet these targets. The Global Burden of Disease (GBD) program has highlighted overweight/obesity as a key issue in global health and dietary risks as one of the top several risk factors for the global burden of disease in low- and middle-income countries (Institute for Health Metrics and Evaluation 2016).[1] And two commissions—the *Lancet* Commission on Obesity and the EAT *Lancet* Commission—released new reports in January 2019, highlighting the catastrophic impacts of overweight/obesity on health and sustainable development (EAT *Lancet* Commission 2019; LCO 2019). A third report from the *Lancet* Commission on the double burden of malnutrition was released in December 2019 (Popkin, Corvalan, and Grummer-Strawn 2019). The LCO report focuses on the syndemic of obesity, undernutrition, and climate change—and double- and triple-duty actions across all sectors that have the potential to address this syndemic. The EAT *Lancet* Commission report focuses primarily on food systems and their impact on nutrition (both undernutrition and overweight/obesity) as well as on climate change. The *Lancet* Commission report on the double burden (undernutrition and overweight) will focus primarily on the epidemiology of the burden and double-duty policy actions. The 2019 State of the World's Children report (UNICEF 2019) also focused on childhood obesity.

Global parliamentarians met in Rome at the Second International Conference on Nutrition in 2014 and noted that food system solutions are needed to address the global scourge of unhealthy diets (FAO and WHO 2018). In countries as diverse as all the small countries of the Caribbean Community (CARICOM) region, most Latin American countries, South Africa, Thailand, Malaysia, many Middle Eastern nations, and the Western Pacific Islands, ministers of health and in most cases prime ministers have noted that overweight/obesity and the related consequences represent the major preventable causes of poor health and increased health care costs. Recognition of the problem is slowly growing in many low- and middle-income countries, but global action that promotes healthy diets and major shifts in food systems is slow.

All of the above commissions and reports are complementary and highlight the need for concerted action across sectors (health, education, agriculture, trade, macroeconomics, and so on) to address this agenda. Despite the fact that the World Bank Group is uniquely positioned to work across these sectors and use the innovative investment and policy instruments at its disposal, the World Bank's investments in this space are still modest at best. This is true across the board: in the health sector and in food systems, trade, fiscal policies, and transport as well as education. The World Bank Group's new *World Development Report* (World Bank 2019) on the future of work does not address the scourge of overweight/obesity and its potential impacts on productivity.

Healthy diets, along with adequate growth in stature and weight, are critical for optimal cognitive development and learning in children. These links to cognitive development, along with the positive health effects of healthy diets and healthy weight, are also critical for improved productivity and reduced disability throughout the life cycle. Healthy diets have profound effects on carbon emissions and water use globally (EAT *Lancet* Commission 2019; Springmann et al. 2018).

The authors hope that this report will spur action among both client countries and development partners such as the World Bank to invest in evidence-based strategies and actions across sectors to address obesity and NCDs.

Last—but perhaps most important—this report hopes to serve as a wake-up call. The time to act is now. The data presented in the report show the enormous and rapidly growing global public health burden of overweight and obesity, but they also suggest that there is still an opportunity to intervene, preventing obesity among adults and children under five—in all countries, not just in low- and middle-income ones. But the opportunity to act is now, before this bomb explodes. The World Bank has just launched a major corporate initiative on building human capital, alongside the release of a new Human Capital Index (HCI) that includes detailed information for 157 countries.[2] The launch of the index has generated the concern and momentum it was intended to among national leaders and ministries of finance in client countries (World Bank 2018b). The HCI focuses on three main ingredients. The third ingredient, health, has two parts: one looks at children's stunting; the other at adult survival rates (ASRs). This focus on adult survival provides a perfect entry point for scaling up country engagement on obesity prevention in order to reduce NCDs and related adult mortality (figure 1.1).

What Is New in This Report?

This report complements all of the new and forthcoming technical reports on overweight/obesity prevention in four distinct ways:

- First, it focuses on identifying evidence-based opportunities for fiscal and regulatory policy reforms and investments across several sectors that could prevent overweight/obesity. In doing so, it builds on the

Figure 1.1 Human Capital Index and Its Links to Nutrition

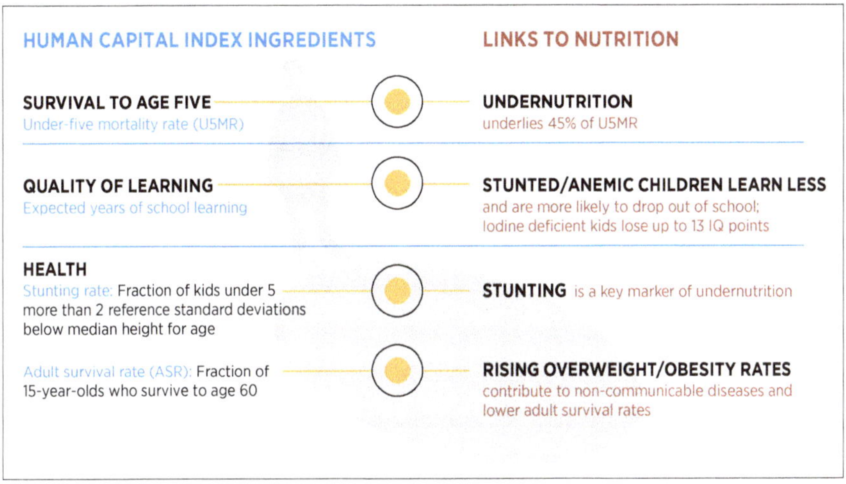

HUMAN CAPITAL INDEX INGREDIENTS	LINKS TO NUTRITION
SURVIVAL TO AGE FIVE Under-five mortality rate (U5MR)	**UNDERNUTRITION** underlies 45% of U5MR
QUALITY OF LEARNING Expected years of school learning	**STUNTED/ANEMIC CHILDREN LEARN LESS** and are more likely to drop out of school; Iodine deficient kids lose up to 13 IQ points
HEALTH Stunting rate: Fraction of kids under 5 more than 2 reference standard deviations below median height for age	**STUNTING** is a key marker of undernutrition
Adult survival rate (ASR): Fraction of 15-year-olds who survive to age 60	**RISING OVERWEIGHT/OBESITY RATES** contribute to non-communicable diseases and lower adult survival rates

Source: Based on World Bank 2018a.

epidemiological evidence from the technical reports; adds new information on the economic implications of overweight/obesity, including the equity perspective; and identifies the growing list of double-burden countries to spur urgent action in these countries.

• Second, it brings to bear implementation challenges and lessons learned from several country case studies where policies or interventions addressing overweight/obesity have been rolled out at scale, with variable success.

• Third, and perhaps most important, it identifies an action agenda that is specifically geared to the unique role that institutions such as the World Bank can play in this space as well as the instruments (including policy and regulatory levers, technical assistance, and results-based financing instruments as well as investment lending) that these institutions can use in the near future to address the emerging epidemic of obesity and related NCDs across sectors.

• Last, the report reiterates research findings from recent technical reports from the *Lancet* that suggest that changing diets and food systems are also key to addressing the ongoing challenge of child stunting/undernutrition, along with the growing challenges of climate change. It identifies key areas requiring further research and evaluations that may be important for building the knowledge base for future actions in this area.

Notes

1. See Global Burden of Disease http://www.healthdata.org/gbd.
2. For information about the Human Capital Project, see http://www.worldbank
   .org/en/publication/human-capital#_blank.

References

Barrientos-Gutierrez, T., R. Zepeda-Tello, E. R. Rodrigues, A. Colchero-Aragonés, R. Rojas-Martínez, E. Lazcano-Ponce, M. Hernández-Ávila, J. Rivera-Dommarco, and R. Meza. 2017. "Expected Population Weight and Diabetes Impact of the 1-Peso-per-Litre Tax to Sugar Sweetened Beverages in Mexico." *PLOS ONE* 12 (5): e0176336.

Constantino-Toto, R. M., and D. Montero. 2016. "Water Footprint of Bottled Drinks and Food Security." In *Water, Food and Welfare*, edited by R. H. Pérez-Espejo, H. R. Dávila-Ibáñez, and R. M. Constantino-Toto, 229–39. New York: Springer Briefs in Environment, Security, Development and Peace.

EAT *Lancet* Commission. 2019. Willett, W., J. Rockström, B. Loken, M. Springmann, T. Lang, S. Vermeulen, T. Garnett, D. Tilman, F. DeClerck, A. Wood, M. Jonell, M. Clark, L. J. Gordon, J. Fanzo, C. Hawkes, R. Zurayk, J. A. Rivera, W. De Vries, L. Majele Sibanda, A. Afshin, A. Chaudhary, M. Herrero, R. Agustina, F. Branca, A. Lartey, S. Fan, B. Crona, E. Fox, V. Bignet, M. Troell, T. Lindahl, S. Singh, S. E. Cornell, K. Srinath Reddy, S. Narain, S. Nishtar, and C. J. L. Murray. "Food in the Anthropocene: The EAT–*Lancet* Commission on Healthy Diets from Sustainable Food Systems." *The Lancet* 393 (10170): 447–92. https://www.thelancet.com/commissions/EAT.

Ercin, A. E., M. M. Aldaya, and A. Y. Hoekstra. 2011. "Corporate Water Footprint Accounting and Impact Assessment: The Case of the Water Footprint of a Sugar-Containing Carbonated Beverage." *Water Resources Management* 25 (2): 721–41.

FAO and WHO (Food and Agriculture Organization of the United Nations and the World Health Organization). 2018. *The Nutrition Challenge and Food System Solutions*. Rome: FAO and WHO. https://apps.who.int/iris/bitstream/handle/10665/277440/WHO-NMH-NHD-18.10-eng.pdf?ua=1.

GBD 2015 Obesity Collaborators. 2017. "Health Effects of Overweight and Obesity in 195 Countries over 25 Years." *New England Journal of Medicine* 377: 13–27.

Institute for Health Metrics and Evaluation. 2016. *Global Burden of Disease Study 2015 (GBD 2015) Covariates 1980–2015*. Seattle: Institute for Health Metrics and Evaluation (IHME).

Jones-Smith, J. C., P. Gordon-Larsen, A. Siddiqi, and B. M. Popkin. 2011. "Cross-National Comparisons of Time Trends in Overweight Inequality by Socioeconomic Status among Women Using Repeated Cross-Sectional Surveys from 37 Developing Countries, 1989–2007." *American Journal of Epidemiology* 173 (6): 667–75.

———. 2012. "Emerging Disparities in Overweight by Educational Attainment in Chinese Adults (1989–2006)." *International Journal of Obesity* 36 (6): 866–75.

Kosen, S. 2018. "The Economic Burden of Overweight and Obesity Reaches 3% of GDP in Indonesia." *Asia Pathways* blog post, February 2. https://www.asiapathways-adbi.org/2018/02/the-economic-burden-of-overweight-and-obesity-in-indonesia/.

LCO (*Lancet* Commission on Obesity). 2019. Swinburn, B. A., V. I. Kraak, S. Allender, V. J. Atkins, P. I. Baker, J. R. Bogard, H. Brinsden, A. Calvillo, O. De Schutter, R. Devarajan, M. Ezzati, S. Friel, S. Goenka, R. A. Hammond, G. Hastings, C. Hawkes, M. Herrero, P. S. Hovmand, M. Howden, L. M. Jaacks, A. B. Kapetanaki, M. Kasman, H. V. Kuhnlein, S. K. Kumanyika, B. Larijani, T. Lobstein, M. W. Long, V. K. R. Matsudo, S. D. H. Mills, G. Morgan, A. Morshed, P. M. Nece, A. Pan, D. W. Patterson, G. Sacks, M. Shekar, G. L. Simmons, W. Smit, A. Tootee, S. Vandevijvere, W. E. Waterlander, L. Wolfenden, and W. H. Dietz. 2019. "The Global Syndemic of Obesity, Undernutrition, and Climate Change: The *Lancet* Commission Report." *The Lancet* 393 (10173): 791–846. https://www.thelancet.com/commissions/global-syndemic.

Lehnert, T., P. Streltchenia, A. Konnopka, S. G. Riedel-Heller, and H. Konig. 2015. "Health Burden and Costs of Obesity and Overweight in Germany: An Update." *European Journal of Health Economics* 16: 957–67.

Popkin, B. M., C. Corvalan, and L. Grummer-Strawn. 2019. "Dynamics of the Double Burden of Malnutrition and the Changing Nutrition Reality." *The Lancet*. https://doi.org/10.1016/S0140-6736(19)32497-3.

Popkin, B. M., S. Kim, E. R. Rusev, S. Du, and C. Zizza. 2006. "Measuring the Full Economic Costs of Diet, Physical Activity and Obesity-Related Chronic Diseases." *Obesity Reviews* 7: 271–93.

Qin, X., and J. Pan. 2016. "The Medical Cost Attributable to Obesity and Overweight in China: Estimation Based on Longitudinal Surveys." *Health Economics* 25 (10): 1291–311.

Rtveladze, K., T. Marsh, L. Webber, F. Kilpi, D. Levy, W. Conde, K. McPherson, and M. Brown. 2013. "Health and Economic Burden of Obesity in Brazil." *PLOS ONE* 8 (7): e68785.

Sánchez-Romero, L. M., J. Penko, P. G. Coxson, A. Fernández, A. Mason, A. E. Moran, L. Ávila-Burgos, M. Odden, S. Barquera, and K. Bibbins-Domingo. 2016. "Projected Impact of Mexico's Sugar-Sweetened Beverage Tax Policy on Diabetes and Cardiovascular Disease: A Modeling Study." *PLOS Medicine* 13 (11): e1002158.

Springmann, M., M. Clark, D. Mason-D-Croz, K. Wiebe, B. L. Bodirsky, L. Lassaletta, W. de Vries, S. J. Vermeulen, M. Herrero, K. M. Carlson, M. Jonell, M. Troell, F. DeClerck, L. J. Gordon, R. Zurayk, P. Scarborough, M. Rayner, B. Loken, J. Fanzo, H. C. J. Godfray, D. Tilman, J. Rockström, and W. Willett. 2018. "Options for Keeping the Food System within Environmental Limits." *Nature* 562 (7728): 519–25.

Trogdon, J. G., E. A. Finkelstein, T. Hylands, P. S. Dellea, and S. J. Kamal-Bahl. 2008. "Indirect Costs of Obesity: A Review of the Current Literature." *Obesity Reviews* 9 (5): 489–500.

UNICEF (United Nations Children's Fund). 2019. *The State of the World's Children. Children, Food and Nutrition: Growing well in a Changing World.* UNICEF, New York.

WHO (World Health Organization). 2013. *Global Action Plan for the Prevention and Control of Noncommunicable Diseases 2013–2020.* Geneva: WHO.

———. 2014a. Global Nutrition Targets 2025: Policy Brief Series (WHO/NMH /NHD/14.2). WHO. https://www.who.int/nutrition/global-target-2025/en/.

———. 2014b. "Global Nutrition Targets 2025: Childhood Overweight." Policy Brief. WHO, Geneva. https://apps.who.int/iris/bitstream/handle/10665/149021 /WHO_NMH_NHD_14.6_eng.pdf?ua=1.

World Bank. 2018a. *The Human Capital Project.* World Bank, Washington, DC. https://openknowledge.worldbank.org/handle/10986/30498. License: CC BY 3.0 IGO.

———. 2018b. "If Countries Act Now, Children Born Today Could Be Healthier, Wealthier, More Productive." Press Release, October 11.

———. 2019. *World Development Report: The Changing Nature of Work.* Washington, DC: World Bank. doi:10.1596/978-1-4648-1328-3. License: Creative Commons Attribution CC BY 3.0 IGO.

2

Prevalence and Trends

Julia Dayton Eberwein, Vanessa Oddo, Jonathan Kweku Akuoku, Kyoko Shibata Okamura, Barry Popkin, and Meera Shekar

---

Key Messages

- In 2016, globally more than two out of five adults (44 percent, or more than 2 billion) and one out of five children ages 5–19 were overweight/obese. Over 70 percent of them lived in low- or middle-income countries, dispelling the myth that overweight/obesity is a problem only in high-income countries.
- Between 1980 and 2016, levels of overweight/obesity increased in all regions of the world. Furthermore, there is increasing evidence that the use of the current body mass index (BMI) cutoff of 25 underestimates the total burden of overweight/obesity in low- and middle-income countries, so the problem may be even more acute than is presented in the global literature.
- Within countries, the burden of overweight/obesity shifts toward the poor as country per capita income increases. In middle-income countries, the poor are just as likely or more likely to be overweight/obese, whereas among low-income countries, overweight/obesity is mainly concentrated among wealthier groups.
- The rapid increases in overweight/obesity in low- and middle-income countries have meant that rural areas across low- and middle-income countries are catching up on overall measures of overweight/obesity with urban areas. The exception is South Asia and most of Sub-Saharan Africa, where overweight/obesity remains primarily an urban phenomenon.

- Over 70 percent of countries—the vast majority of which are low- and lower-middle-income ones—currently face a double burden: high prevalence of both undernutrition and overweight/obesity. High levels of the double burden are increasingly found in the poorest low-income countries.

What Is Overweight/Obesity?

Overweight/obesity occurs when excess energy is stored in fat cells. Fat cells enlarge and increase in number, accumulating in the abdominal region, in muscle, and around organs such as the liver, kidneys, pancreas, and heart. This proliferation of fat cells produces numerous metabolic, hormonal, and inflammatory chemicals that adversely affect the body's arteries, tissues, and organ functions. The inflammatory and metabolic changes to body processes result in high cholesterol, high blood pressure, insulin resistance, and high blood glucose, which together can develop into non-communicable diseases (NCDs) such as diabetes, cardiovascular disease, and cancer (Esser et al. 2014; GBD 2015 Obesity Collaborators 2017; WCRF and AICR 2018). Physiological changes lead to stress on joints, impaired ability to move, and breathing problems such as shortness of breath and sleep apnea. The resulting lack of sleep, stress, and impaired ability to be physically active (as occurs with osteoarthritis) further exacerbate weight gain (Felson et al. 1988; Patel and Hu 2008).

Global Overweight/Obesity Prevalence

Worldwide, an estimated 44 percent of adults and 20 percent of children over five years of age are either overweight or obese, hereafter referred to as *overweight/obese*. Overweight and obesity are measured using BMI.

Overweight/obesity has nearly tripled since 1975 and now accounts for 4 million deaths globally every year, nearly two-thirds of which are due to cardiovascular disease; it also accounts for approximately 120 million lost disability-adjusted life years (DALYs) (GBD 2015 Obesity Collaborators 2017). Once considered a public health problem only in high-income countries, overweight/obesity is now highly prevalent in low- and middle-income countries. Consequently, low- and middle-income countries are now confronted with the *double burden of malnutrition*, characteristically defined by the coexistence of undernutrition and overweight/obesity (Dietz 2017).

This chapter presents trends in overweight/obesity prevalence globally and by region, gender, and age based on repeated cross-sectional ecological data from two data sources: (1) the NCD Risk Factor Collaboration Study (NCD-RisC 2019) for adults and children ages five years and older,[1] and (2) the Joint Child Malnutrition Estimates (JME) for children under five years of age (UNICEF, WHO, and World Bank 2016).[2]

In 2016, approximately 6 percent of children under 5, 20 percent of children ages 5–19, and 44 percent of adults ages 20 years and older were overweight or obese (figure 2.1). There are no significant gender differences among children under 5, but boys 5–19 are more likely to be overweight/obese than girls of the same age. Among adults, the prevalence of overweight/obesity is higher among men (29 percent) than women (25 percent); however, 19 percent of women are overweight/obese as compared with 15 percent of men.

Figure 2.2 shows the distribution of overweight/obese individuals across country income groups. In all age groups, the majority of overweight/obese individuals reside in middle-income countries, dispelling the myth that overweight/obesity is a problem only in high-income countries.

Cutoffs of public health significance have long been established for various dimensions of undernutrition such as stunting, wasting, underweight, and anemia (WHO 2011, 2012; WHO Multicentre Growth Reference Study Group 2006); these have proven useful in describing the severity of the

Figure 2.1 Global Overweight and Obesity Rates: Children under 5 and Ages 5–19, and Adults Ages 20+

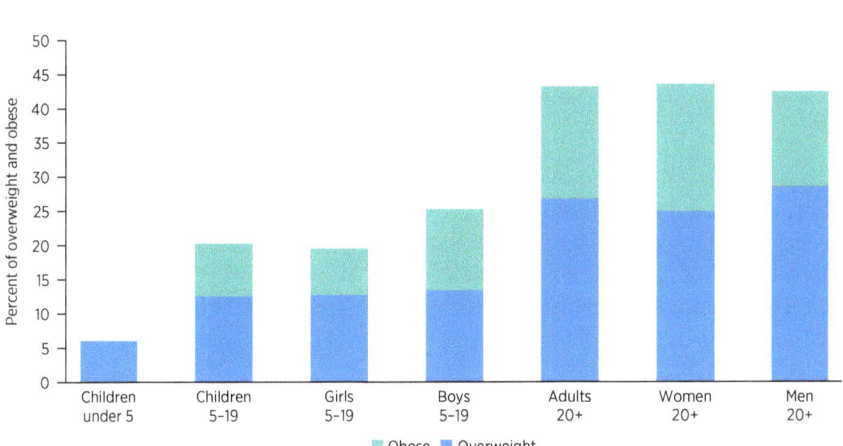

Sources: Data for children under 5 are from UNICEF, WHO, and World Bank 2016; data for adults are from NCD-RisC estimates for 2016, http://ncdrisc.org/data-downloads.html.

Figure 2.2 More Than Three-Quarters of Overweight/Obese Individuals Live in Middle-Income Countries

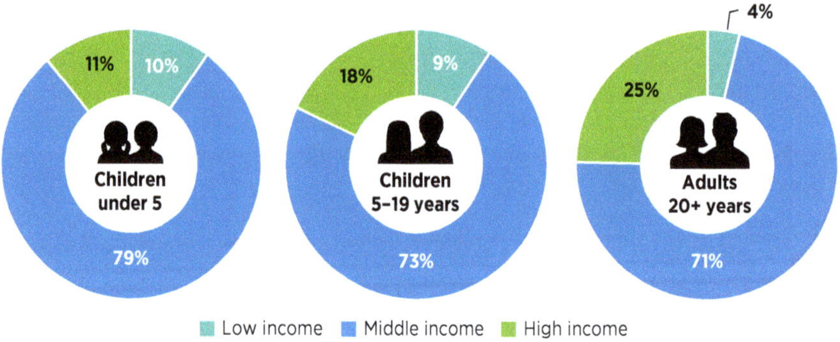

Sources: Data on overweight and obesity levels from NCD-RisC estimates for 2016, http://ncdrisc.org/data-downloads.html; country income classifications based on World Bank criteria as of 2015.

Table 2.1 Proposed Cutoff Values for Public Health Significance of Country-Level Double Burden of Malnutrition

Overweight/obesity prevalence in adults	Stunting prevalence in children under 5			
	≥ 30%	20–29%	10–19%	< 10%
≥40%	Very high	High	Moderate	Low or none
30–39%	High	High	Moderate	Low or none
20–29%	Moderate	Moderate	Moderate	Low or none
< 20%	Low or none	Low or none	Low or none	Low or none

Sources: Stunting cutoffs are defined using WHO Multicentre Growth Reference Study Group 2006; overweight/obesity cutoffs are based on original recommendations and Popkin, Corvalan, and Grummer-Strawn 2019.

problem across time and place and as an important impetus for public action. There are, however, currently no existing global cutoffs for determining the public health significance of overweight/obesity at the country level. To date the World Health Organization (WHO) and United Nations Children's Fund (UNICEF) have established cutoffs for countries for levels of underweight and stunting, but not for overweight. In table 2A.1, the chapter authors propose cutoffs for adults, adolescents, and children in order to identify countries facing a critical prevalence of overweight/obesity. These cutoffs for adults are the same as those in the forthcoming *Lancet* report on the double burden of undernutrition and overweight (Popkin, Corvalan, and Grummer-Strawn 2019), which recommends cutoffs of 19, 20 to 29, 30 to 39, and

≥ 40 percent prevalence for determining severe overweight/obesity among adult subpopulations (see table 2.1).

When viewed by age group (map 2.1), the data for 2016 show that although public health significance levels seem relatively lower for children under 5 (panel a), the public health significance of overweight/obesity becomes high and very high among older children and adults (as shown in

Map 2.1 **Proposed Public Health Significance of Overweight/Obesity by Age and Country**

a. Children under 5

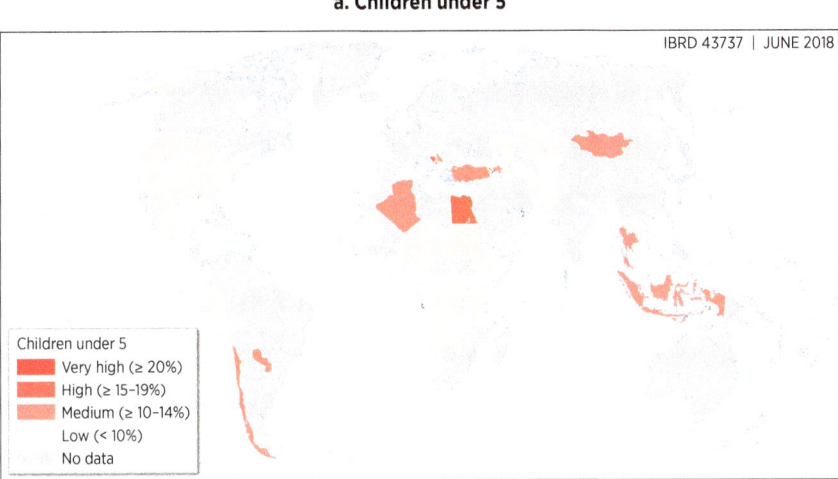

b. Children Ages 5–19

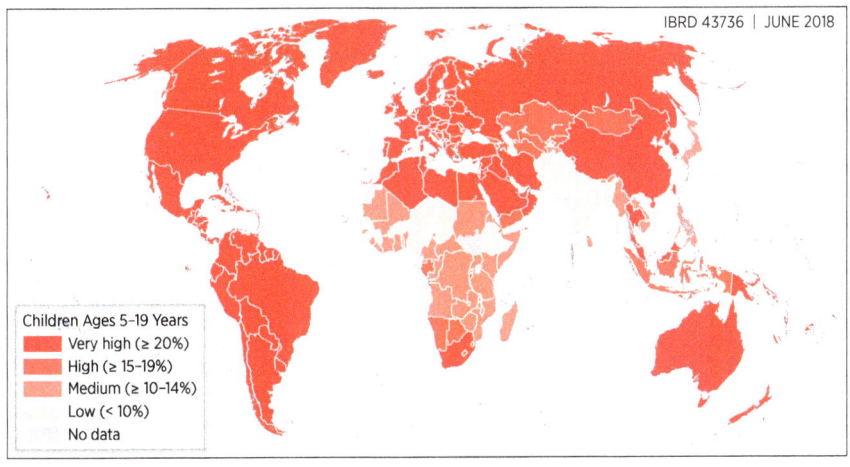

continued next page

Map 2.1 *(continued)*

c. Adults Ages 20+

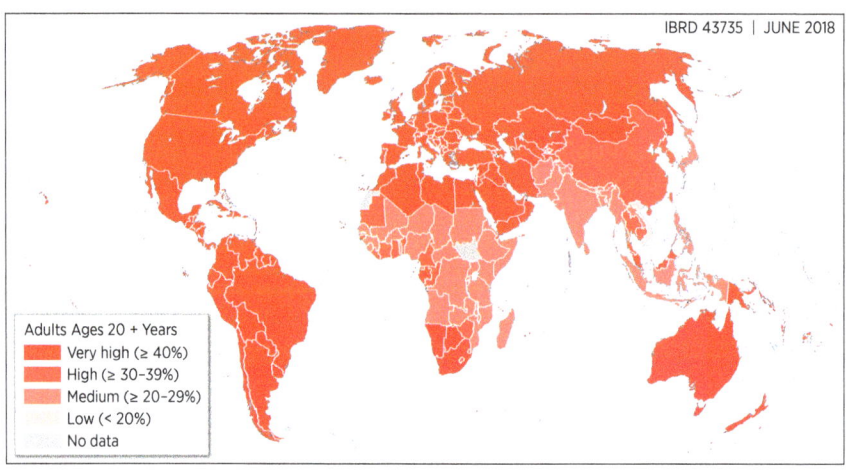

Source: NCD-RisC estimates for 2016, http://ncdrisc.org/data-downloads.html.

panels b and c). In most countries, fewer than 10 percent of children under 5 are overweight/obese, but some countries have high rates of overweight/obesity among children 5–19 and adults. These data show the enormous global public health burden of overweight and obesity, but they also suggest that there is still an opportunity to intervene and prevent overweight/obesity among children under 5, particularly in low- and middle-income countries. But the opportunity to act is now, before this time bomb explodes.

Global and Regional Trends in Overweight/Obesity over Time

Between 1980 and 2016, prevalence rates of overweight/obesity increased dramatically in all regions of the world (see map 2.2) and in all age groups (see figure 2.3). The prevalence of overweight is higher than the prevalence of obesity, but the increase over time in obesity prevalence (not shown) is greater.

In all countries with high adult overweight/obesity levels that began in the 1990s, there was a lag of about seven years or more before child and adolescent overweight/obesity also accelerated, as shown in figure 2.3. Latin America, North Africa, and South East and East Asia, among other regions, are beginning to show higher prevalence of child/adolescent over-weight and the rates of change are accelerating.

Although these trends are alarming in and of themselves, it is impor-tant to note that these estimates of overweight/obesity prevalence ignore one critical issue. There is increasing evidence that using a BMI cutoff of 25 underestimates the total burden of overweight/obesity in

Map 2.2   Overweight/Obesity Prevalence by Country Income Level

a. Low- and Middle-Income Countries

1990s

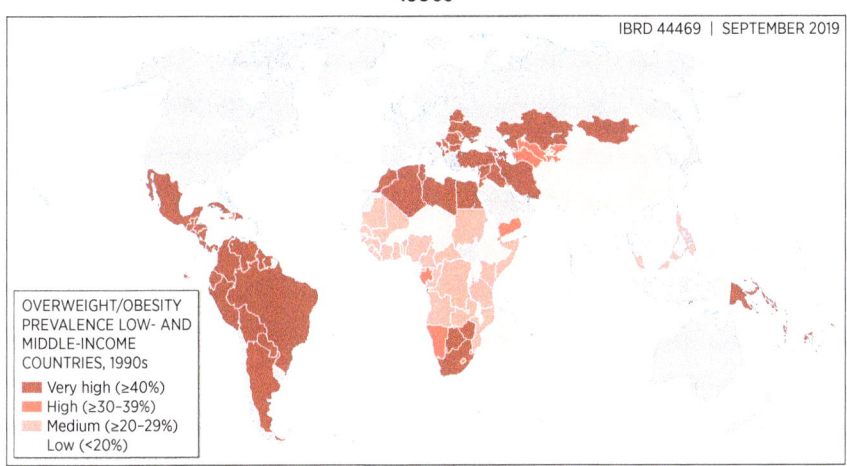

2010s

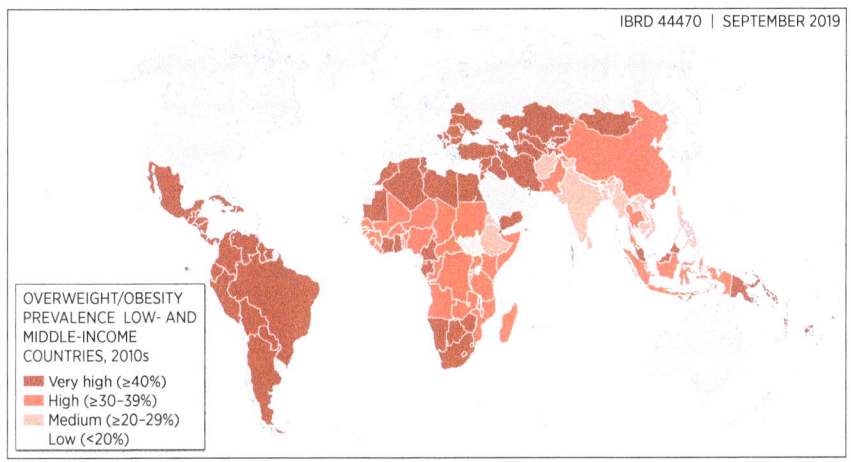

continued next page

Map 2.2 *(continued)*

b. High-Income Countries
1990s

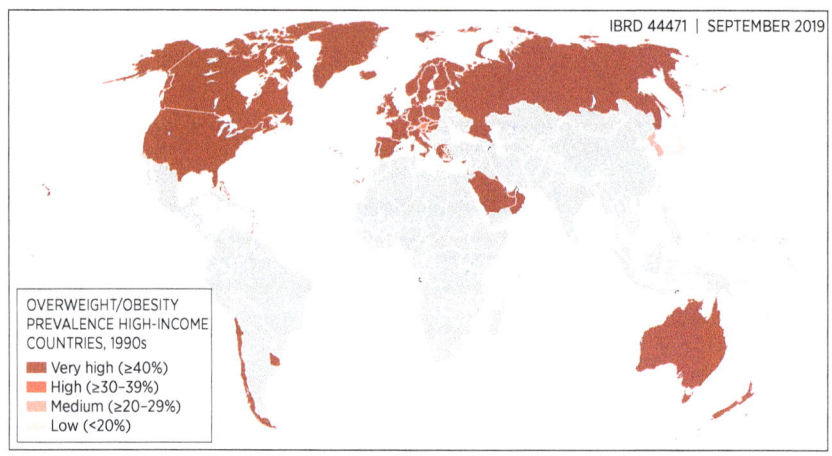

2010s

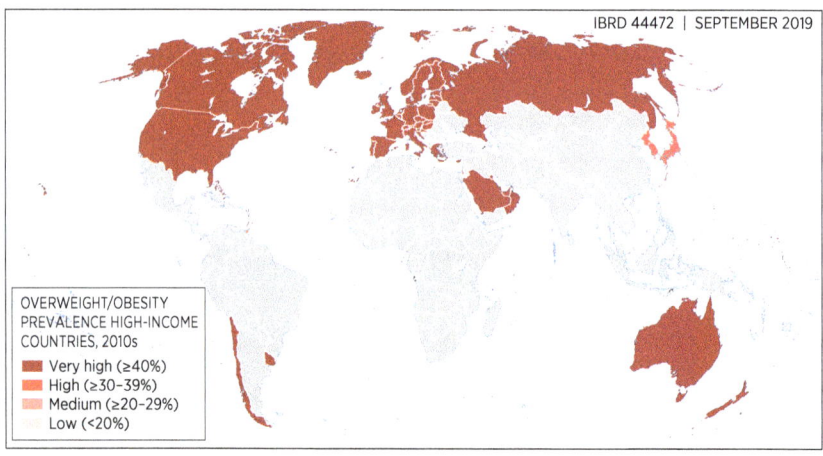

Sources: Popkin, Global Food Research Program, University of North Carolina. Data are from UNICEF, WHO, World Bank, and NCD-RisC estimates, supplemented with selected Demographic and Health Surveys and other country direct national measures.

Note: Based on 1990s and 2010s weight and height data.

Figure 2.3 Prevalence of Overweight/Obesity by Age Group and Region, 1980–2016

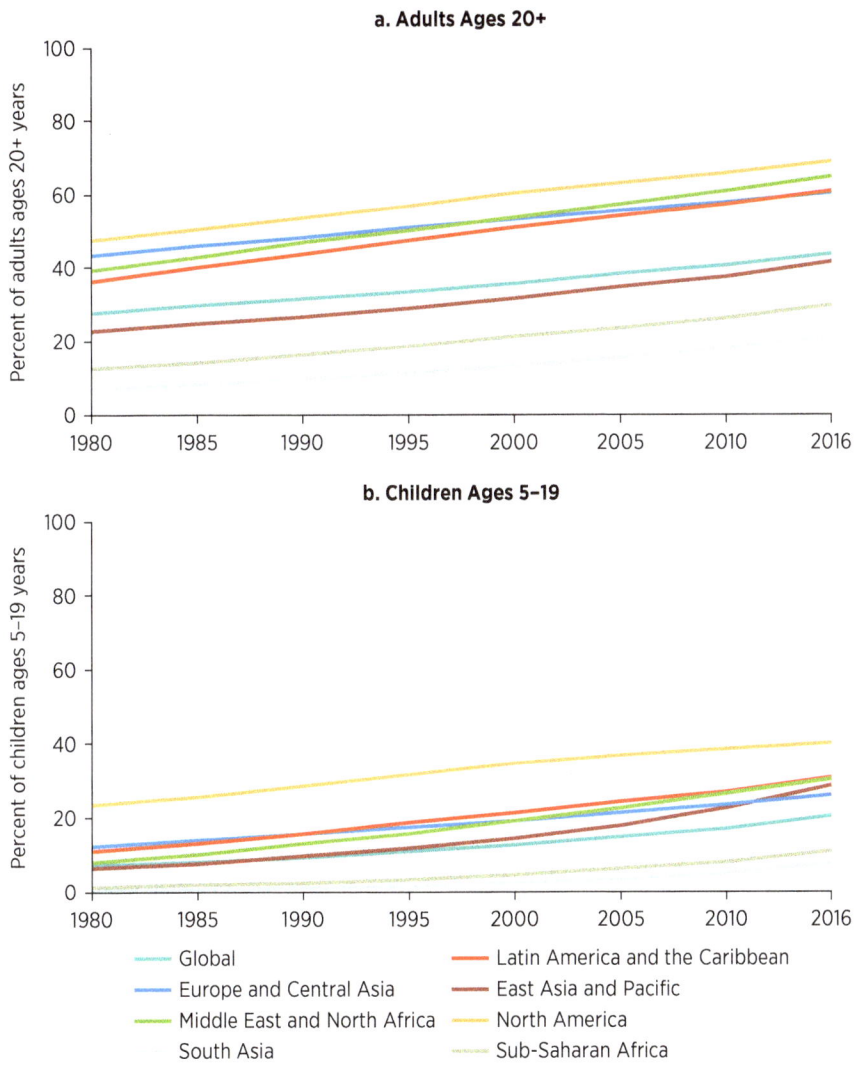

a. Adults Ages 20+

b. Children Ages 5–19

Global
Europe and Central Asia
Middle East and North Africa
South Asia
Latin America and the Caribbean
East Asia and Pacific
North America
Sub-Saharan Africa

continued next page

Figure 2.3 *(continued)*

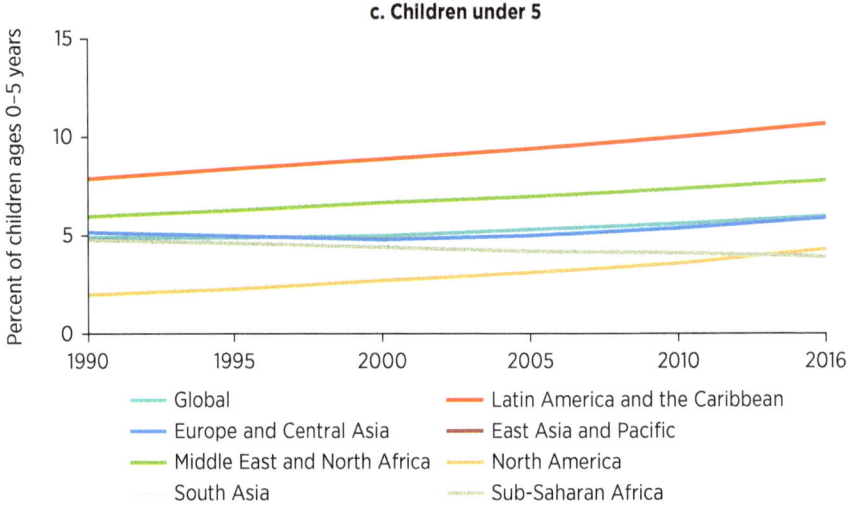

c. Children under 5

Sources: Data for children under 5 are from UNICEF, WHO, and World Bank 2016; data for children ages 5–19 and adults are from NCD-RisC estimates for 2016, http://ncdrisc.org/data-downloads.html.

low- and middle-income countries. There is a large push in Asia and selected other regions to lower the BMI cutoff for overweight to 25 because most major subpopulation groups (for example, Asians, Hispanics from Mexico south to Chile in the Andean region, Africans) experience increased risks of diabetes and hypertension at much lower BMI levels. One regional WHO-International Obesity Task Force meeting and subsequent work from China advocated for a lower overweight and obesity cutoff of a BMI level of 23 and 28, respectively (WHO Expert Consultation 2004). Studies in Latin America and Asia have shown larger comparative risks of hypertension and diabetes at much lower levels of BMI than among non-Hispanic whites (Albrecht, Mayer-Davis, and Popkin 2017; Bell, Adair, and Popkin 2002; WHO Expert Consultation 2004). This is also the case for South Asians with very high proportions of visceral fat (body fat around the heart and liver, also sometimes called *visceral adiposity* or *central adiposity*) and increased risks of diabetes at BMI levels of 22–23 (Wells et al. 2016). Many studies comparing South Asians to other population subgroups replicate these results (Joshi et al. 2007; Misra 2015; Nair and Prabhakaran 2012).

The Equity Perspective

The sections below consider overweight/obesity prevalence by socioeconomic status and by urban/rural groups to provide a context for ensuring equity in the global approach to the problem.

Overweight/Obesity Prevalence by Income Group within Countries

Although the national-level data reported in this chapter do not allow for describing overweight/obesity rates by income group within a given country, evidence from Demographic and Health Surveys (DHS) from selected low- and middle-income countries suggests that, as country income increases, the burden of overweight/obesity shifts from the wealthy to the poor (figure 2.4) (Jones-Smith et al. 2011, 2012b). Today in most countries in Latin America, the Middle East, Eastern Europe, Central Asia, and East Asia (specifically China and Indonesia), there are now more overweight/obese individuals among the poor, lower socioeconomic status population than among higher income and higher socioeconomic status populations. This is not the case in either South Asia or Sub-Saharan Africa. These two regions have increasing proportions of overweight/obesity but also still have the bulk of the stunted populations of the world and the highest prevalence of a double burden of malnutrition (Popkin, Corvalan, and Grummer-Strawn 2019). The only country with both a severe level of double burden and greater overweight/obesity among the poor is Indonesia.

The crossover to higher rates of overweight/obesity among poorer income groups as country income increases is not entirely captured in the selection of countries included in the DHS (Popkin, Corvalan, and Grummer-Strawn, forthcoming). However, empirical evidence from Brazil (Monteiro et al. 2000; Monteiro, Conde, and Popkin 2001, 2007) and China (Jones-Smith et al. 2012a) shows a greater burden of overweight/ obesity among the poor/lower socioeconomic status. Similar results are reported for Indonesia and Sub-Saharan Africa (Aizawa and Helble 2016; Ziraba, Fotso, and Ochako 2009). Furthermore, Jones-Smith et al. (2011; 2012a) also show that the prevalence of overweight/obesity has increased more quickly over time for the poorest (versus wealthiest) women in a number of low- and middle-income countries.[3]

One review that analyzes the association between household income and obesity in children shows that obesity among children and adolescents is more prevalent among the affluent in low- and middle-income countries, suggesting that the shift in obesity in children from wealthier to

Figure 2.4   Shift in Burden of Overweight/Obesity to the Poor
GNI per capita, US$

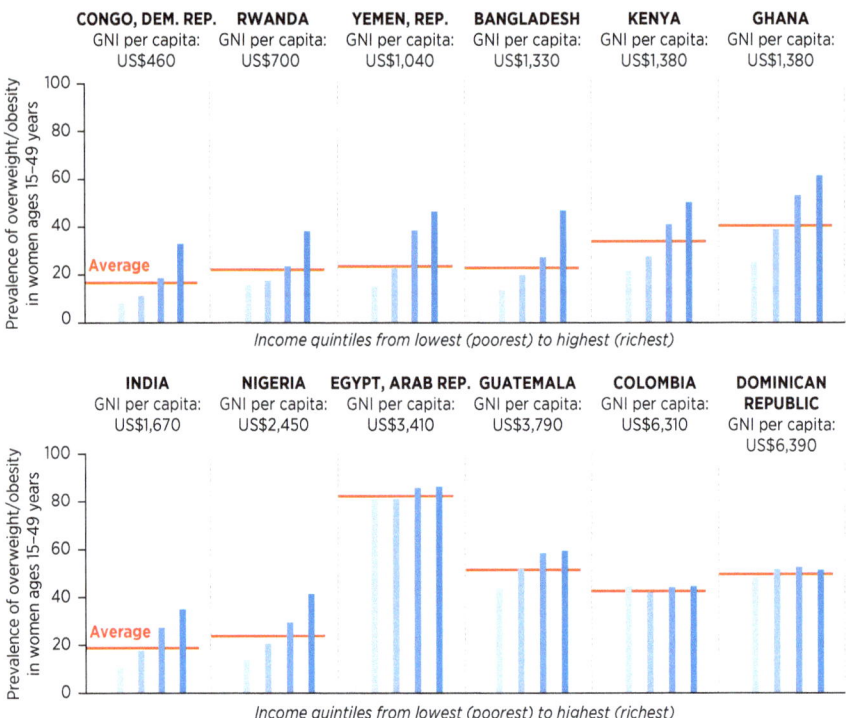

Sources: Demographic and Health Surveys from Democratic Republic of Congo 2013, Rwanda 2014, Republic of Yemen 2013, Kenya 2014, Ghana 2014, India 2015, Nigeria 2013, Arab Republic of Egypt 2014, Guatemala 2014, Colombia 2010, Dominican Republic 2013; https://dhsprogram.com/What-We-Do/Survey-Search.cfm/.

Note: GNI = gross national income.

poorer segments of the population may occur at a higher level of national income than it does for adults (Dinsa et al. 2012).[4] However, further analyses specifically addressing this question among children in low- and middle-income countries are urgently needed.

Overweight/Obesity Rates by Urban/Rural Residence within Countries

Previous analyses have demonstrated higher rates of overweight/obesity in urban than in rural residents within a country, particularly in low-income countries that are in earlier phases of their nutrition transition (Jaacks, Slining, and Popkin 2015; Mendez, Monteiro, and Popkin 2005).

Figure 2.5 Prevalence of Overweight/Obesity among Women Ages 15–49 by Urban/Rural Residence, Selected Low- and Middle-Income Countries

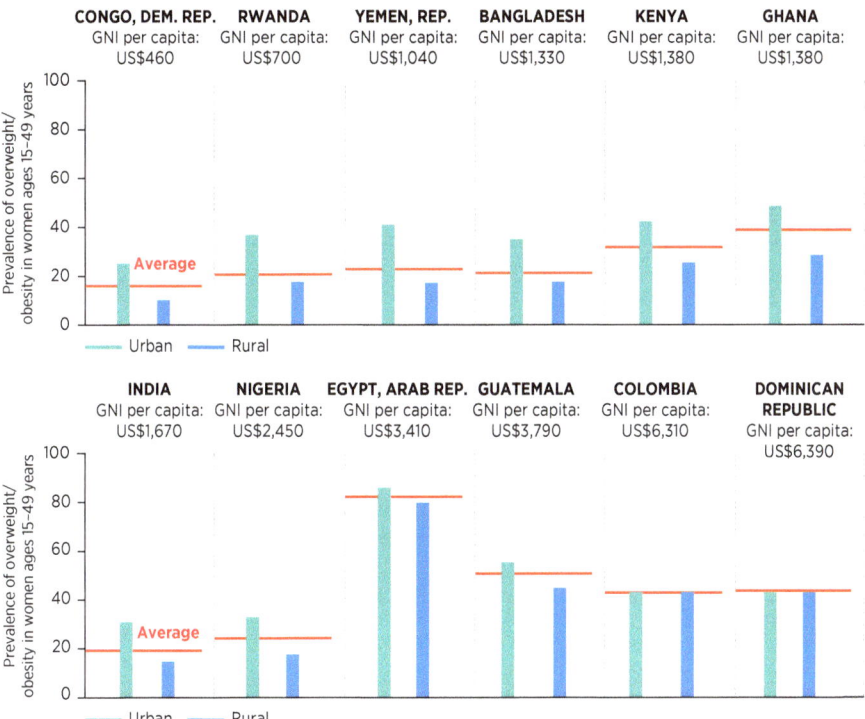

Sources: Demographic and Health Surveys from Democratic Republic of Congo 2013, Rwanda 2014, Republic of Yemen 2013, Kenya 2014, Ghana 2014, India 2015, Nigeria 2013, Arab Republic of Egypt 2014, Guatemala 2014, Colombia 2010, Dominican Republic 2013; https://dhsprogram.com/What-We-Do/Survey-Search.cfm/.

Note: GNI = gross national income.

However, DHS results from selected low- and middle-income countries show that overweight/obesity is not exclusive to urban areas. (As previously stated, national-level data do not allow for describing overweight/ obesity prevalence by urban/rural residence.) The panels in figure 2.5 show the prevalence of overweight/obesity by area of residence among women, with countries ordered from lowest to highest GNI per capita. The Sub-Saharan African and South Asian countries are where the proportion of overweight/obesity is much greater in urban areas. Among lower-income countries, the prevalence of overweight/obesity among women is considerably higher in urban areas. However, the prevalence of overweight/obesity is still high—approximately 20 percent—even in rural areas. In higher-income countries (for example, in upper-middle-income countries), overweight/obesity prevalence is more equally distributed across women living in urban and rural areas, dispelling the common misconception that the overweight/obesity burden is limited to urban areas. There is also evidence that the prevalence of overweight/obesity is increasing faster now in many rural areas among lower-income countries (Jaacks, Slining, and Popkin 2015). Greater overweight/obesity in rural areas is expected by 2025 in all regions of the world except Sub-Saharan Africa.

This implies that a future focus on rural as well as urban overweight/obesity will be required and represents a major shift in thinking for much of the world—in high-income countries, middle-income countries, and low-income ones.

The Double Burden of Malnutrition

This section first defines exactly what is meant by the *double burden of malnutrition* and considers how this double burden can be analyzed and described at multiple levels. It then identifies countries that experience particularly high double burdens and, finally, considers trends over time.

Definition

The *double burden of malnutrition* (hereafter referred to as the *double burden*), defined as concurrent burdens of overweight and undernutrition (WHO 2017), is hypothesized to be driven by increased economic development and the concurrent nutrition transition that leads to changes in food and physical activity patterns (Ng and Popkin 2012; Popkin 2004; Shrimpton and Rokx 2012).

The double burden can be analyzed and described at individual, household/community, and national levels, and within a population of adults, children, or a combination of the two (Abdullah 2015; Doak et al. 2000; Doak et al. 2002; Doak et al. 2005; Garrett and Ruel 2005; Popkin, Corvalan, and Grummer-Strawn 2019). For this report, the double burden is defined with respect to population-level prevalence of overnutrition among adult women and prevalence of undernutrition among children under five. There are two primary reasons for this choice. First, the double burden is driven largely by increasing rates of overweight/obesity as undernutrition recedes or stagnates during the nutrition transition. Changes in food systems (production, marketing, consumption), urbanization, modern technology, and the built environment are key factors for the increasing prevalence of overweight/obesity; these are amenable to change through national-level policy making and interventions. Second, there are established guidelines for assessing the public health significance of undernutrition, as characterized by stunting, at the country level based on the recently revised thresholds by de Onis et al. (2018). This report proposes new cutoffs for the public health significance of overweight/obesity (see table 2.1 for proposed cutoff values). Using the established cutoff guidelines for stunting and this report's proposed cutoffs for overweight/obesity, this report classifies countries according to the level of double burden.

Countries Identified by WHO Undernutrition Criteria as Having Severe Levels of Double Burden

Today most of the countries in the world with high levels of the double burden are found in Sub-Saharan Africa, South Asia, South East Asia (Indonesia being the most prominent), plus Guatemala. This is a marked shift from the 1990s, when Mexico and most of Central America, Bolivia, and Peru, South Africa, Francophone Africa, the Arab Republic of Egypt, parts of Central Asia, and the Philippines faced severe levels of the double burden. Map 2.3 shows this dramatic shift.

Figures 2.6–2.11 present countries in each region by plotting their level of the double burden of malnutrition, consisting of prevalence of childhood stunting and overweight/obesity among women. Generally, stunting prevalence is inversely related to women's overweight/obesity prevalence. However, significant clusters of countries experience medium or high levels of the double burden. Guatemala, Papua New Guinea, and the Republic of Yemen have very high double burdens, with child stunting prevalence above 40 percent alongside adult female overweight/obesity in excess of 50 percent. Botswana, Cameroon, Djibouti, Lesotho, and the Solomon Islands also have high levels of double burden, with stunting prevalence above 30 percent and overweight/obesity prevalence ranging between 41 percent and 62 percent. The largest high-double-burden country is Indonesia, with about 36 percent stunting and over 40 percent female overweight/obesity.

Prevalence of the double burden varies widely by region (figures 2.6 through 2.11 and figure 2A.1; country-level double burden is presented in table 2A.2; the level of double burden by country income group is shown in figures 2A.2 through 2A.5). Using the metric established in this report, most countries with a double burden are in Sub-Saharan Africa, with a significant majority of countries experiencing a medium to high double burden. Of the 48 Sub-Saharan Africa countries included, 46 (96 percent) have a medium to very high double burden.

Map 2.3 Double Burden of Malnutrition: Low- and Middle-Income Countries

a. 1990s

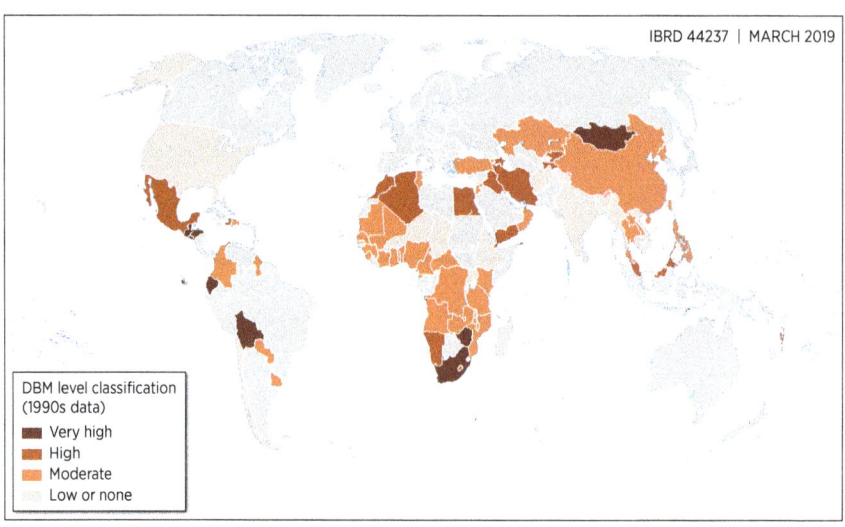

b. 2010s

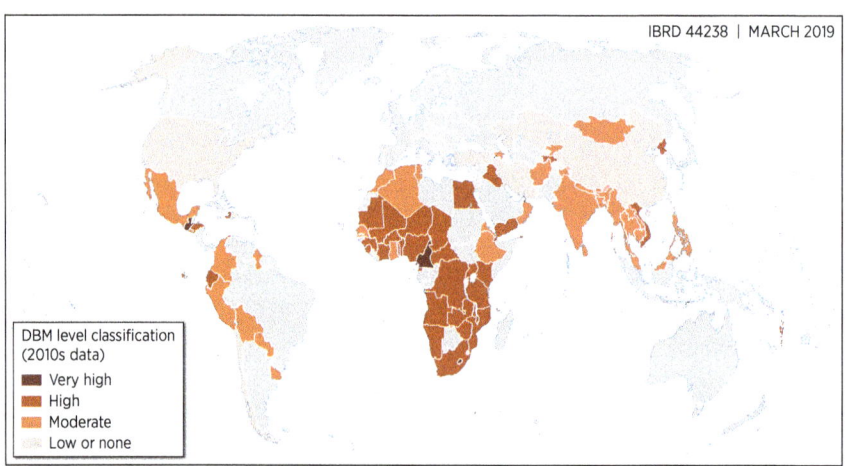

Sources: Data from Joint Child Malnutrition Estimates (UNICEF, WHO, World Bank) and NCD-RisC estimates; country income classifications based on World Bank criteria as of 2015.

Figure 2.6 Country-Level Double Burden of Malnutrition, East Asia and Pacific

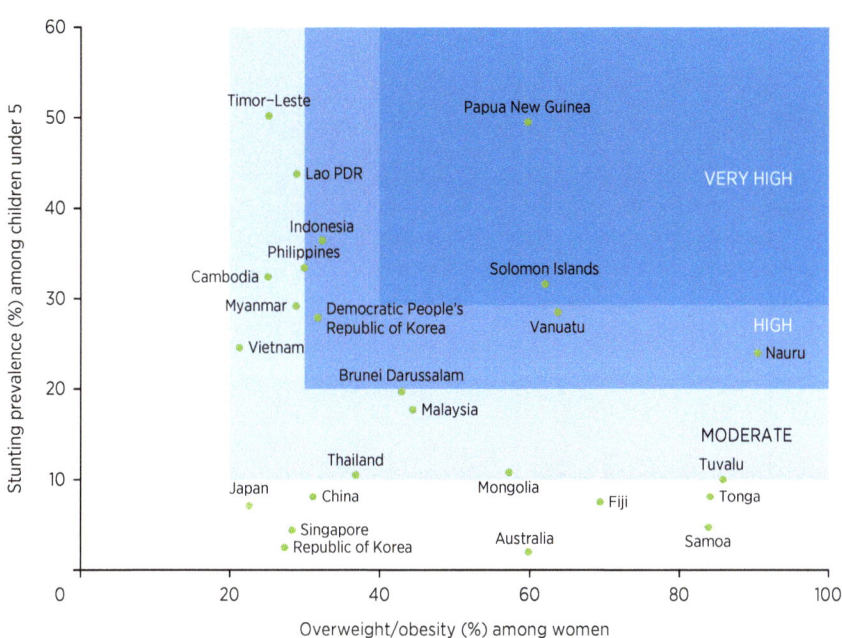

Sources: Data for stunting prevalence are from UNICEF, WHO, and World Bank 2016; data for overweight/obesity are from NCD-RisC estimates for 2016, http://ncdrisc.org/data-downloads.html.

In East Asia and Pacific, 17 of the 26 countries have medium to very high double burdens, driven mainly by the high prevalence of stunting and medium prevalence of overweight/obesity. Papua New Guinea has a very high double burden, with very high stunting prevalence (50 percent) and very high overweight/obesity (60 percent). In countries without a double burden, rates of overweight/obesity are alarming, with the majority ranging between 40 percent and more than 80 percent.

The forthcoming *Lancet* series on the double burden will show that increasingly it is the low-income countries that have the greatest double burden (Popkin, Corvalan, and Grummer-Strawn 2019).

Trends in the Double Burden over Time

Overall, most low- and middle-income countries have experienced declines in stunting prevalence but they invariably show rising

Figure 2.7 Country-Level Double Burden of Malnutrition, Europe and Central Asia

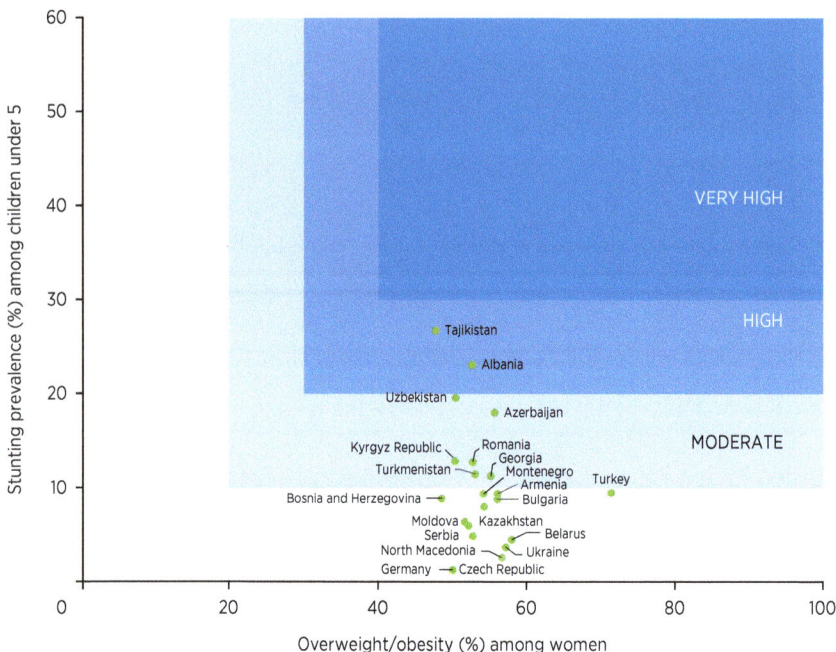

Sources: Data for stunting prevalence are from UNICEF, WHO, and World Bank 2016; data for overweight/obesity are from NCD-RisC estimates for 2016, http://ncdrisc.org/data-downloads.html.

prevalence of overweight/obesity. Thus, countries have progressed from having a high stunting burden only to have a double burden, with reduced but still high prevalence of stunting along with increased prevalence of overweight/obesity. In a few countries, stunting prevalence stagnated or increased while overweight/obesity prevalence increased. When all lower-middle-income countries in the 1990s were stratified by current gross national product per capita using World Bank purchasing power parity levels, countries from the 1990s that are now in the middle- and higher-income group (but were classified as low-income countries in the 1990s) had significantly reduced their likelihood of being a double-burden country.

Over time, the lower-income countries have been much more likely to become high-double-burden countries (map 2.3). This is once again indicative of the spread of overweight/obesity to lower-middle-income countries, the rapid growth in consumption of unhealthy foods and beverages, and

Figure 2.8 Country-Level Double Burden of Malnutrition, Latin America and the Caribbean

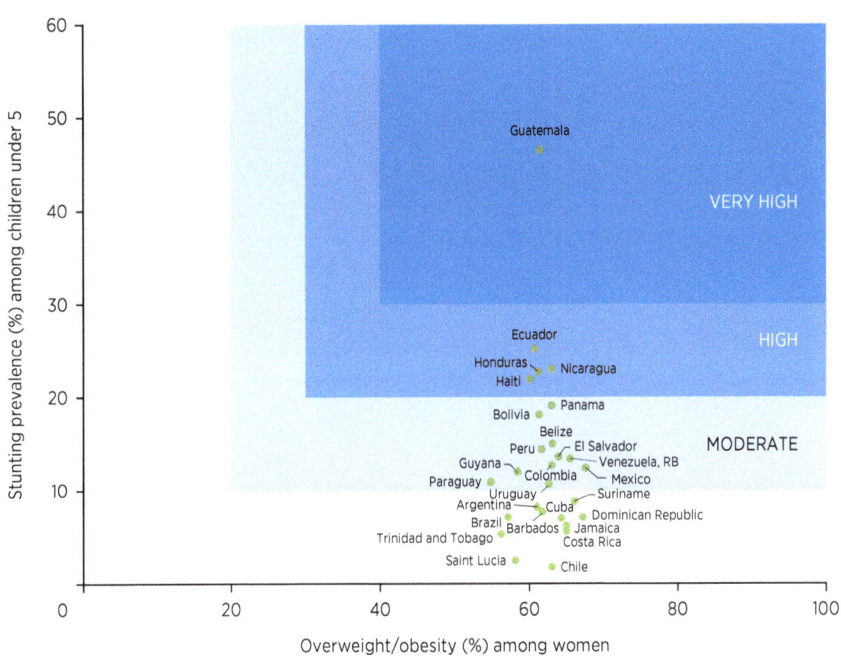

Sources: Data for stunting prevalence are from UNICEF, WHO, and World Bank 2016; data for overweight/obesity are from NCD-RisC estimates for 2016, http://ncdrisc.org/data-downloads.html.

the remarkable shifts in technology, which affect activity globally (Popkin, Corvalan, and Grummer-Strawn 2019; Pries et at. 2019).

It is important to note that there is a considerable lag between stunting during the preschool period and subsequent NCD complications. A large established literature on the way stunting in early childhood affects subsequent visceral fat increases and the risks of many NCDs exists (Adair et al. 2013; Kuzawa et al. 2012; Stein et al. 2010; Victora et al. 2008; Wells, Wibaek, and Poullas 2018). Levels of stunting in the 1990s, for example, will be reflected right now only among those in the 20- to 30-year-old age group. Clearly there is a lag, as shown by a set of long-term birth cohort studies on the consequences of rises in visceral fat (the type of overweight with greater risks of NCDs) both because of these critical biological causes and because of the reduced energy expenditure and changing food patterns discussed in the next two chapters (Adair et al. 2013; Stein et al. 2010; Victora et al. 2008). This literature suggests that

Figure 2.9   Country-Level Double Burden of Malnutrition, Middle East and North Africa

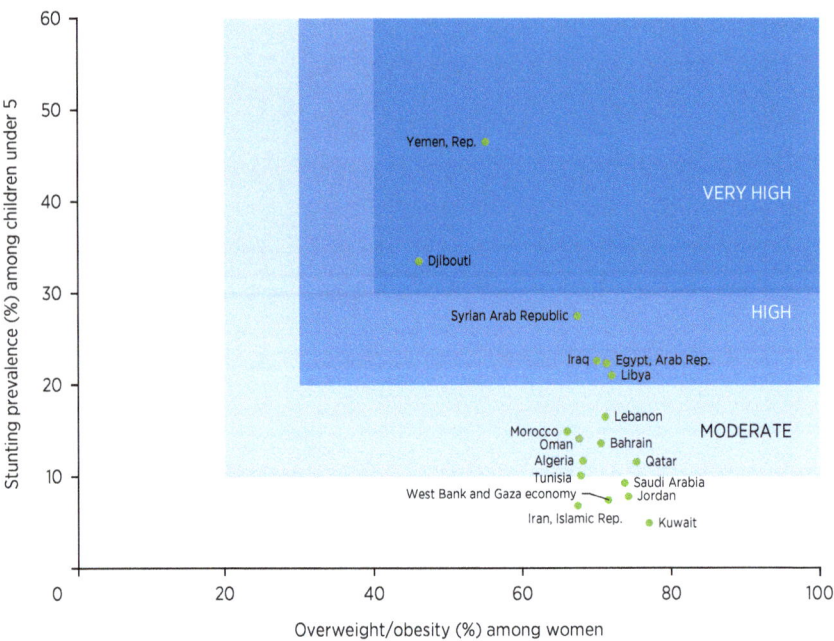

Sources: Data for stunting prevalence are from UNICEF, WHO, and World Bank 2016; data for overweight/obesity are from NCD-RisC estimates for 2016, http://ncdrisc.org/data-downloads.html.

the coming generations of young adults as well as current older adults will experience an increased risk of NCDs at lower BMI levels since they were stunted during the vulnerable first 1,000 days. Furthermore, continued intergenerational problems that lead to excessive low birthweight among infants, increased risk of stunted and subsequently overweight/obese adults, and other adverse outcomes are expected for several future decades based on past and current levels of stunting (Wells et al., forthcoming; Wells, Wibaek, and Poullas 2018). Programs to reduce child stunting are therefore one way to prevent future increased risks of many overweight/obesity-related NCDs. The following chapters lay out some of the potential actions that can prevent overweight/obesity.

Figure 2.10   Country-Level Double Burden of Malnutrition, South Asia

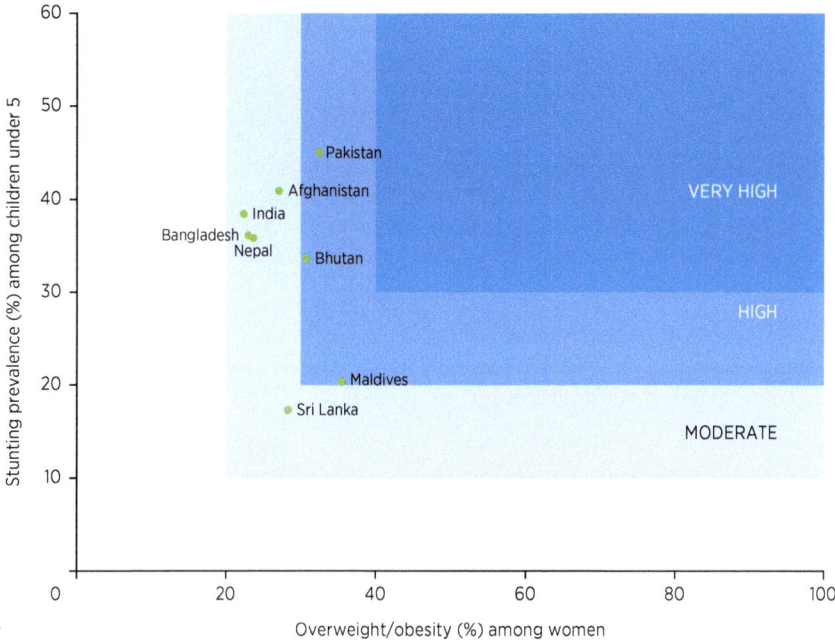

Sources: Data for stunting prevalence are from UNICEF, WHO, and World Bank 2016; data for overweight/obesity are from NCD-RisC estimates for 2016, http://ncdrisc.org /data-downloads.html.

Figure 2.11   Country-Level Double Burden of Malnutrition, Sub-Saharan Africa

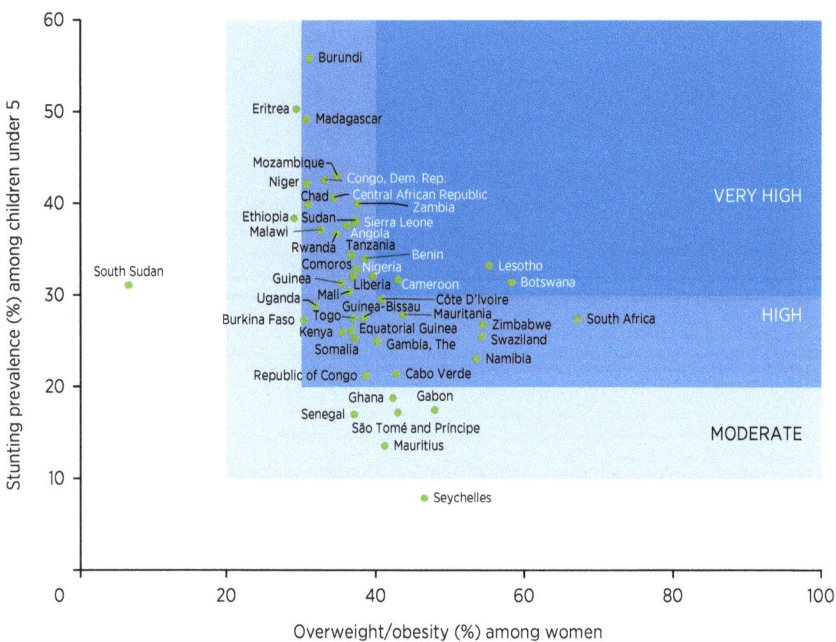

Sources: Data for stunting prevalence are from UNICEF, WHO, and World Bank 2016; data for overweight/obesity are from NCD-RisC estimates for 2016, http://ncdrisc.org /data-downloads.html.

Annex 2A: Prevalence of Overweight/Obesity: Additional Tables and Figures

Table 2A.1 Proposed Cutoff Values for Public Health Significance of Prevalence of Overweight/Obesity, Adults and Children

Prevalence group	Prevalence of overweight/obesity	Global		Low-income countries		Middle-income countries		High-income countries	
		Number of countries	Percent	Number of countries	Percent	Number of countries	Percent	Number of countries	Percent
Adults ages 20 and older									
Low	< 20%	1	1	0	0	1	1	0	0
Medium	≥ 20–29%	41	21	23	77	17	16	1	2
High	≥ 30–39%	23	12	6	20	14	13	3	5
Very high	≥ 40%	129	66	1	3	75	70	53	93
Total		194		30		107		57	
Children ages 5–19 years[a]									
Low	< 10%	13	7	8	27	5	5	0	0
Medium	≥ 10–14%	42	22	20	67	21	20	1	2
High	≥ 15–19%	18	9	0	0	18	17	0	0
Very high	≥ 20%	121	62	2	7	63	59	56	98
Total		194		30		107		57	
Children under 5 years[b]									
Low	< 10%	67	80	20	95	44	77	3	50
Medium	≥ 10–14%	13	15	1	5	9	16	3	50
High	≥ 15–19%	3	4	0	0	3	5	0	0
Very high	≥ 20%	1	1	0	0	1	2	0	0
Total		84		21		57		6	

a. NCD-RisC does not disaggregate children by age; however, it may be preferable to generate cutoffs separately for adolescents ages 15–19, particularly girls since they have likely undergone menarche.

b. Estimated using Joint Child Malnutrition Estimates (JME) data between 2011 and 2016. Where multiple years of data are available, overweight/obesity prevalence is averaged across time periods.

Figure 2A.1 Prevalence of Overweight/Obesity by Region

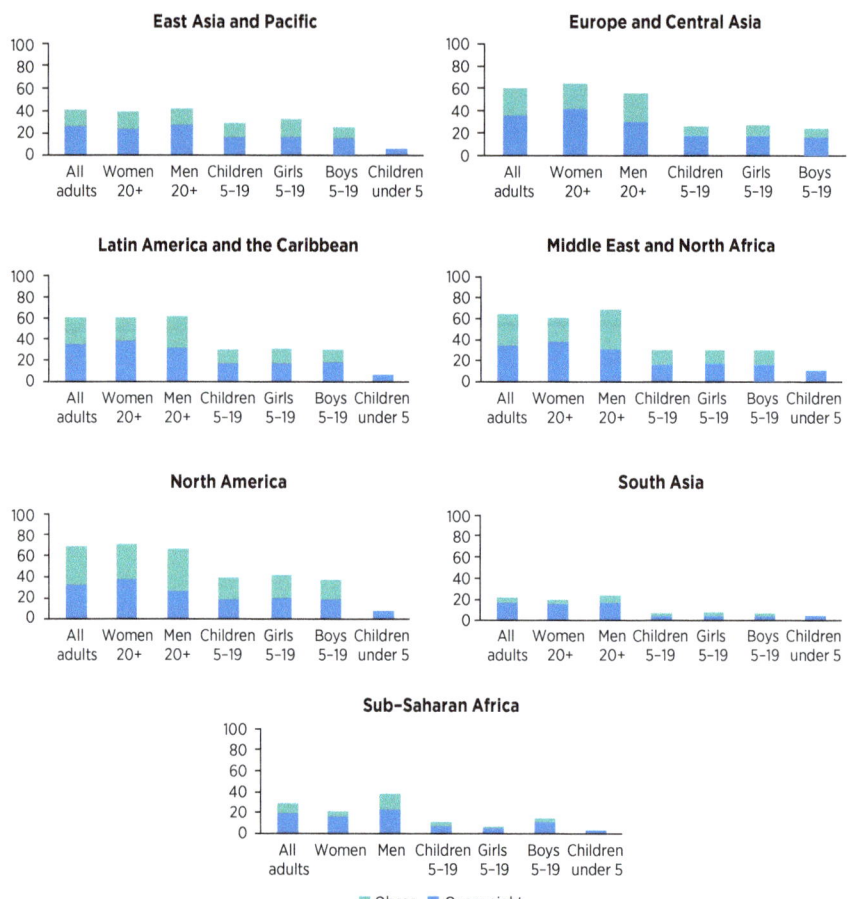

Sources: Data for adults and children 5–19 are from NCD-RisC estimates for 2016, http://ncdrisc.org/data-downloads.html; data for children under 5 are from UNICEF, WHO, and World Bank 2016, Joint Child Malnutrition Estimates, https://www.who.int/nutgrowthdb/estimates2016/en/, accessed July 2017.

Table 2A.2   Level of Double Burden by Country

Country/economy	Income group	Stunting prevalence (%, children under 5)	Overweight/ obesity (%, women)	Level of double burden
East Asia and Pacific				
Australia	High income	2.0	59.8	Low or none
Brunei Darussalam	High income	19.7	42.9	Moderate
Cambodia	Lower-middle income	32.4	25.1	Moderate
China	Upper-middle income	8.1	31.1	Low or none
Fiji	Upper-middle income	7.5	69.4	Low or none
Indonesia	Lower-middle income	36.4	32.3	High
Japan	High income	7.1	22.6	Low or none
Kiribati	Lower-middle income	—	82.9	Low or none
Korea, Dem. Peoples' Rep.	Low income	27.9	31.7	High
Korea, Rep.	High income	2.5	27.3	Low or none
Lao PDR	Lower-middle income	43.8	28.9	Moderate
Malaysia	Upper-middle income	17.7	44.4	Moderate
Mongolia	Lower-middle income	10.8	57.2	Moderate
Myanmar	Lower-middle income	29.2	28.8	Moderate
Nauru	Upper-middle income	24.0	90.3	High
Papua New Guinea	Lower-middle income	49.5	59.7	Very high
Philippines	Lower-middle income	33.4	29.9	Moderate
Samoa	Upper-middle income	4.7	83.8	Low or none
Singapore	High income	4.4	28.3	Low or none
Solomon Islands	Lower-middle income	31.6	62.0	Very high
Thailand	Upper-middle income	10.5	36.8	Moderate
Timor-Leste	Lower-middle income	50.2	25.2	Moderate
Tonga	Upper-middle income	8.1	84.0	Low or none
Tuvalu	Upper-middle income	10.0	85.7	Moderate
Vanuatu	Lower-middle income	28.5	63.7	High
Vietnam	Lower-middle income	24.6	21.3	Moderate

continued next page

53

Country/economy	Income group	Stunting prevalence (%, children under 5)	Overweight/ obesity (%, women)	Level of double burden
Europe and Central Asia				
Albania	Upper-middle income	23.1	52.7	High
Armenia	Lower-middle income	9.4	56.1	Low or none
Azerbaijan	Upper-middle income	18.0	55.7	Moderate
Belarus	Upper-middle income	4.5	58.0	Low or none
Bosnia and Herzegovina	Upper-middle income	8.9	48.6	Low or none
Bulgaria	Upper-middle income	8.8	56.1	Low or none
Czech Republic	High income	2.6	56.7	Low or none
Georgia	Lower-middle income	11.3	55.2	Moderate
Germany	High income	1.3	50.1	Low or none
Kazakhstan	Upper-middle income	8.0	54.3	Low or none
Kyrgyz Republic	Lower-middle income	12.9	50.4	Moderate
Moldova	Lower-middle income	6.4	51.7	Low or none
Montenegro	Upper-middle income	9.4	54.2	Low or none
North Macedonia	Upper-middle income	4.9	52.8	Low or none
Romania	Upper-middle income	12.8	52.8	Moderate
Serbia	Upper-middle income	6.0	52.2	Low or none
Tajikistan	Lower-middle income	26.8	47.8	High
Turkey	Upper-middle income	9.5	71.4	Low or none
Turkmenistan	Upper-middle income	11.5	53.1	Moderate
Ukraine	Lower-middle income	3.7	57.2	Low or none
Uzbekistan	Lower-middle income	19.6	50.5	Moderate
Latin America and the Caribbean				
Argentina	Upper-middle income	8.2	61.0	Low or none
Barbados	High income	7.7	61.7	Low or none
Belize	Upper-middle income	15.0	63.1	Moderate
Bolivia	Lower-middle income	18.1	61.3	Moderate
Brazil	Upper-middle income	7.1	57.1	Low or none
Chile	High income	1.8	63.0	Low or none
Colombia	Upper-middle income	12.7	63.0	Moderate
Costa Rica	Upper-middle income	5.6	65.0	Low or none

continued next page

Country/economy	Income group	Stunting prevalence (%, children under 5)	Overweight/ obesity (%, women)	Level of double burden
Cuba	Upper-middle income	7.0	64.3	Low or none
Dominican Republic	Upper-middle income	7.1	67.2	Low or none
Ecuador	Upper-middle income	25.2	60.7	High
El Salvador	Lower-middle income	13.6	63.9	Moderate
Guatemala	Lower-middle income	46.5	61.5	Very high
Guyana	Upper-middle income	12.0	58.4	Moderate
Haiti	Low income	21.9	60.1	High
Honduras	Lower-middle income	22.7	61.2	High
Jamaica	Upper-middle income	6.2	65.0	Low or none
Mexico	Upper-middle income	12.4	67.6	Moderate
Nicaragua	Lower-middle income	23.0	63.0	High
Panama	Upper-middle income	19.1	63.0	Moderate
Paraguay	Upper-middle income	10.9	54.8	Moderate
Peru	Upper-middle income	14.4	61.6	Moderate
Saint Lucia	Upper-middle income	2.5	58.1	Low or none
Suriname	Upper-middle income	8.8	66.1	Low or none
Trinidad and Tobago	High income	5.3	56.2	Low or none
Uruguay	High income	10.7	62.6	Moderate
Venezuela, RB	Upper-middle income	13.4	65.5	Moderate
Middle East and North Africa				
Algeria	Upper-middle income	11.7	68.1	Moderate
Bahrain	High income	13.6	70.5	Moderate
Djibouti	Lower-middle income	33.5	46.1	Very high
Egypt, Arab Rep.	Lower-middle income	22.3	71.3	High
Iran, Islamic Rep.	Upper-middle income	6.8	67.4	Low or none
Iraq	Upper-middle income	22.6	70.0	High
Jordan	Lower-middle income	7.8	74.2	Low or none
Kuwait	High income	4.9	77.0	Low or none
Lebanon	Upper-middle income	16.5	71.1	Moderate

continued next page

Country/economy	Income group	Stunting prevalence (%, children under 5)	Overweight/ obesity (%, women)	Level of double burden
Libya	Upper-middle income	21.0	72.0	High
Morocco	Lower-middle income	14.9	66.0	Moderate
Oman	High income	14.1	67.6	Moderate
Qatar	High income	11.6	75.3	Moderate
Saudi Arabia	High income	9.3	73.7	Low or none
Syrian Arab Republic	Lower-middle income	27.5	67.4	High
Tunisia	Lower-middle income	10.1	67.8	Moderate
West Bank and Gaza	Lower-middle income	7.4	71.5	Low or none
Yemen, Rep.	Lower-middle income	46.5	55.1	Very high
North America				
Canada	High income	—	60.1	Low or none
United States	High income	2.1	64.8	Low or none
South Asia				
Afghanistan	Low income	40.9	27.1	Moderate
Bangladesh	Lower-middle income	36.1	23.0	Moderate
Bhutan	Lower-middle income	33.6	30.7	High
India	Lower-middle income	38.4	22.4	Moderate
Maldives	Upper-middle income	20.3	35.4	High
Nepal	Low income	35.8	23.7	Moderate
Pakistan	Lower-middle income	45.0	32.4	High
Sri Lanka	Lower-middle income	17.3	28.3	Moderate
Sub-Saharan Africa				
Angola	Lower-middle income	37.6	36.1	High
Benin	Low income	34.0	38.6	High
Botswana	Upper-middle income	31.4	58.3	Very high
Burkina Faso	Low income	27.3	30.3	High
Burundi	Low income	55.9	31.1	High
Cabo Verde	Lower-middle income	21.4	42.8	High

continued next page

Country/economy	Income group	Stunting prevalence (%, children under 5)	Overweight/ obesity (%, women)	Level of double burden
Cameroon	Lower-middle income	31.7	43.0	Very high
Central African Republic	Low income	40.7	34.4	High
Chad	Low income	39.9	30.9	High
Comoros	Low income	32.1	36.9	High
Congo, Rep.	Lower-middle income	21.2	38.7	High
Côte d'Ivoire	Lower-middle income	29.6	40.8	High
Congo, Dem. Rep.	Low income	42.6	33.2	High
Equatorial Guinea	Upper-middle income	26.2	36.7	High
Eritrea	Low income	50.3	29.3	Moderate
Ethiopia	Low income	38.4	29.0	Moderate
Gabon	Upper-middle income	17.5	48.0	Moderate
Gambia, The	Low income	25.0	40.2	High
Ghana	Lower-middle income	18.8	42.3	Moderate
Guinea	Low income	31.3	35.4	High
Guinea-Bissau	Low income	27.6	38.5	High
Kenya	Lower-middle income	26.0	35.5	High
Lesotho	Lower-middle income	33.2	55.3	Very high
Liberia	Low income	32.1	39.6	High
Madagascar	Low income	49.2	30.7	High
Malawi	Low income	37.1	32.6	High
Mali	Low income	30.4	36.4	High
Mauritania	Lower-middle income	27.9	43.8	High
Mauritius	Upper-middle income	13.6	41.2	Moderate
Mozambique	Low income	43.1	34.8	High
Namibia	Upper-middle income	23.1	53.6	High
Niger	Low income	42.2	30.7	High
Nigeria	Lower-middle income	32.9	37.4	High
Rwanda	Low income	36.7	34.7	High

continued next page

Country/economy	Income group	Stunting prevalence (%, children under 5)	Overweight/ obesity (%, women)	Level of double burden
São Tomé and Príncipe	Lower-middle income	17.2	43.0	Moderate
Senegal	Low income	17.0	37.1	Moderate
Seychelles	High income	7.9	46.6	Low or none
Sierra Leone	Low income	37.9	37.2	High
Somalia	Low income	25.3	37.2	High
South Africa	Upper-middle income	27.4	67.2	High
South Sudan	Low income	31.1	0.0	Low or none
Sudan	Lower-middle income	38.2	37.3	High
Swaziland	Lower-middle income	25.5	54.3	High
Togo	Low income	27.5	37.0	High
Uganda	Low income	28.9	31.9	High
Tanzania	Low income	34.4	36.7	High
Zambia	Lower-middle income	40.0	37.6	High
Zimbabwe	Low income	26.8	54.5	High

Sources: Stunting cutoffs are defined in de Onis et al. (2019), Data for stunting prevalence are from UNICEF, WHO, and World Bank 2016; data for overweight/obesity are from NCD-RisC estimates for 2016, http://ncdrisc.org/data-downloads.html using WHO Multicentre Growth Reference Study Group 2006; overweight/obesity cutoffs are based on original recommendations and Popkin, Corvalan, and Grummer-Strawn 2019.

Note: — = not available.

Figure 2A.2   Country-Level Double Burden: Low-Income Countries

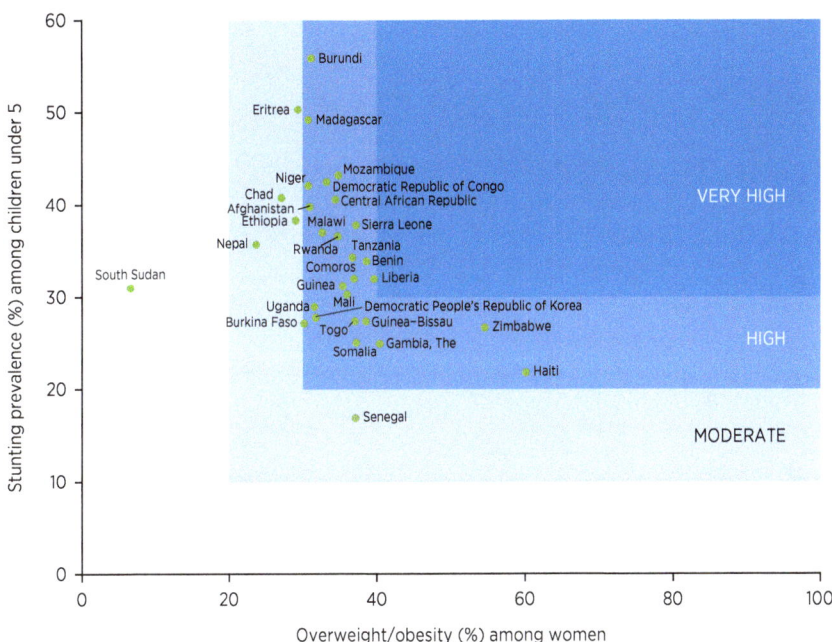

Sources: Data for stunting prevalence are from UNICEF, WHO, and World Bank 2016; data for overweight/obesity are from NCD-RisC estimates for 2016, http://ncdrisc.org /data-downloads.html.

Figure 2A.3 Country-Level Double Burden: Lower-Middle-Income Countries

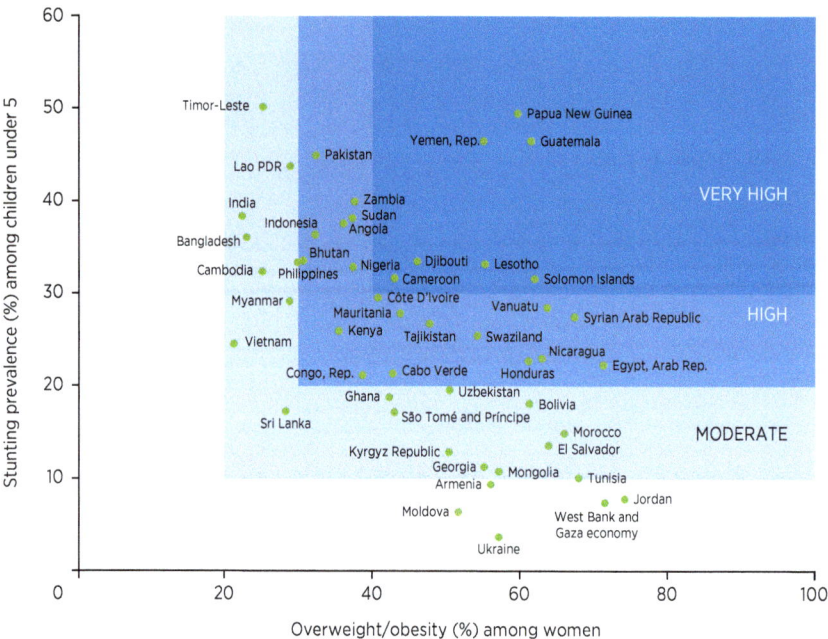

Sources: Data for stunting prevalence are from UNICEF, WHO, and World Bank 2016; data for overweight/obesity are from NCD-RisC estimates for 2016, http://ncdrisc.org /data-downloads.html.

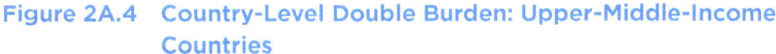

Figure 2A.4   Country-Level Double Burden: Upper-Middle-Income Countries

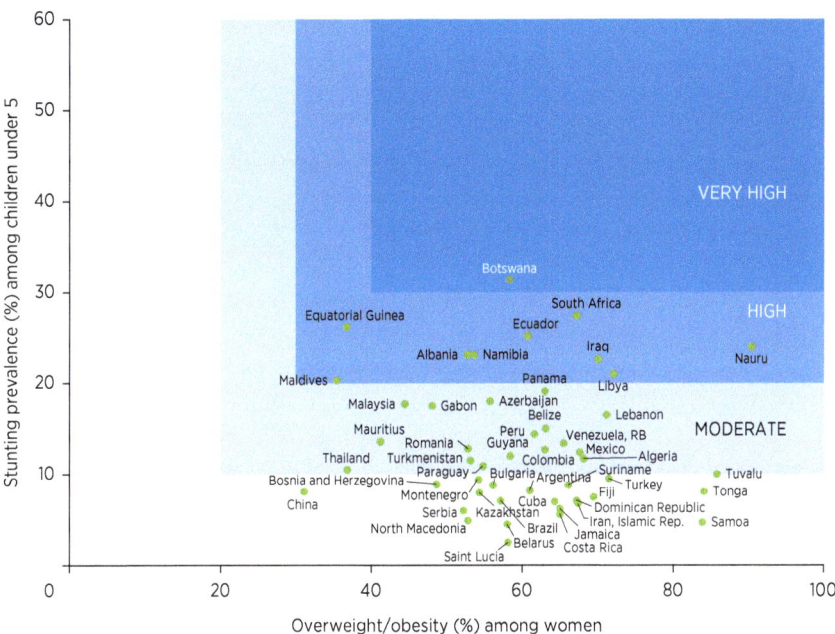

Sources: Data for stunting prevalence are from UNICEF, WHO, and World Bank 2016; data for overweight/obesity are from NCD-RisC estimates for 2016, http://ncdrisc.org /data-downloads.html.

Figure 2A.5 Country-Level Double Burden: High-Income Countries

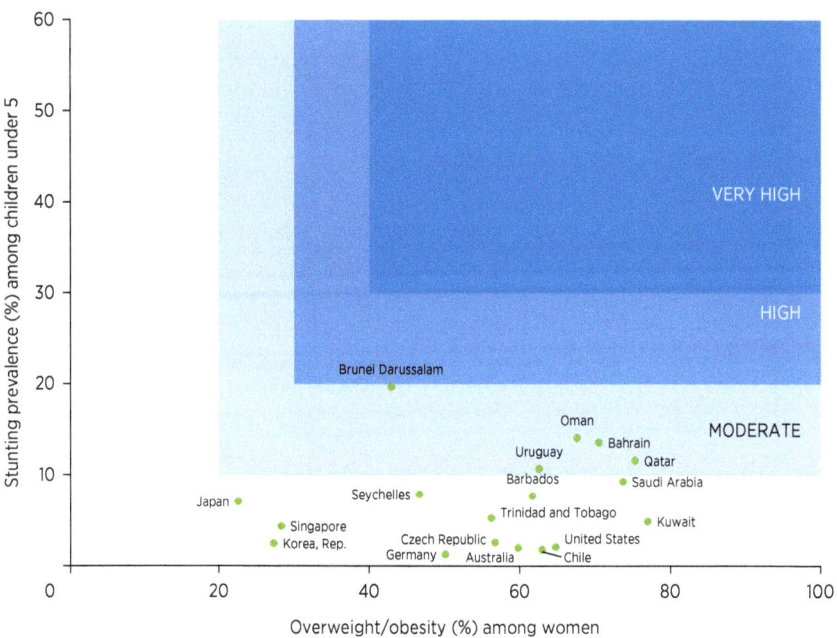

Sources: Data for stunting prevalence are from UNICEF, WHO, and World Bank 2016; data for overweight/obesity are from NCD-RisC estimates for 2016, http://ncdrisc.org /data-downloads.html.

Notes

1. NCD-RisC is coordinated by the WHO Collaborating Centre on NCD Surveillance and Epidemiology and currently has data from over 2,545 population-based surveys from 194 countries from 1975 to 2016 for children ages 5–19 and adults (ages 20 and over). To obtain population-based surveys, NCD-RisC first accessed publicly available population-based multicountry and national measurement surveys (for example, Demographic and Health Surveys [DHS]) and then requested data from (1) ministries of health and other national health agencies to identify population-based surveys and (2) a global network of health researchers. To identify data sources not accessed through the aforementioned mechanisms, researchers also conducted a literature search via Medline. Where possible, data were reanalyzed to estimate mean BMI and overweight and obesity prevalence rates in standard age groups. Participants with implausible BMI levels, defined as BMI < 10 kg/m^2 or BMI > 80 kg/m^2 (<0.2 percent of all subjects), were excluded from estimates. Some estimates are imputed based on the weighted and smoothed residuals from data for neighboring countries. Notably, the NCD-RisC data use measured (not self-reported) weight and height data to create BMI values.

2. Joint Child Malnutrition Estimates (JME) are coordinated by UNICEF, the WHO, and the World Bank Group. In 2017, the JME consisted of data for children under five from 806 national surveys. UNICEF and the WHO receive and review survey data from the published and gray literature on a continual basis. The WHO maintains the WHO Global Database on Child Growth and Malnutrition, a repository of standardized anthropometric child data that has existed for 20 years. UNICEF maintains a global database populated in part through its annual data collection exercise that draws on submissions from more than 150 country offices. Historical survey estimates based on the U.S. National Center for Health Statistics/WHO growth reference, for which no raw data are available, have been converted to WHO-based prevalence rates (that is, 2006 WHO standards).

3. Relatedly, higher GDP per capita and lower income inequality is also associated with disproportionately faster increases in overweight/obesity prevalence for the lower wealth women, compared with higher wealth women, in low- and middle-income countries (Jones-Smith et al. 2011).

4. Dinsa et al. (2012) identified 11 studies that considered children and adolescents in their review of studies covering low- and middle-income countries published between 2004 and 2010. The studies unanimously showed obesity among children and adolescents as being more prevalent among the affluent in low- and middle-income countries. This is in contrast to results from high-income countries, which have generally shown an inverse association with socioeconomic status (particularly education) and have concluded that child obesity is largely a problem of poverty in high-income countries (Hardy et al. 2017; Knai et al. 2012; Watts et al. 2016).

   Hardy et al. (2017) who analyzed trends in child and adolescent obesity in New South Wales, Australia, between 1985 and 2015, found that disparities by socioeconomic status increased over time. Using longitudinal data for a large cohort of adolescents in the United States, Watts et al. (2016) found that the prevalence of overweight/obesity increased significantly from adolescence to young adulthood with a larger increase occurring among those with low socioeconomic status at baseline, as compared with those with high socioeconomic status.

References

Abdullah, A. 2015. "The Double Burden of Undernutrition and Overnutrition in Developing Countries: An Update." *Current Obesity Reports* 4 (3): 337–49.

Adair, L. S., C. H. Fall, C. Osmond, A. D. Stein, R. Martorell, M. Ramirez-Zea, H. S. Sachdev, D. L. Dahly, I. Bas, S. A. Norris, L. Micklesfield, P. Hallal, and C. G. Victora. 2013. "Associations of Linear Growth and Relative Weight Gain during Early Life with Adult Health and Human Capital in Countries of Low and Middle Income: Findings from Five Birth Cohort Studies." *Lancet* 382 (9891): 525–34.

Aizawa, T., and M. Helble. 2016. "Socioeconomic Inequity in Excessive Weight in Indonesia." ADBI Working Paper 572. Asian Development Bank Institute, Tokyo. https://www.adb.org/sites/default/files/publication/183799/adbi-wp572.pdf.

Albrecht, S. S., E. Mayer-Davis, and B. M. Popkin. 2017. "Secular and Race/Ethnic Trends in Glycemic Outcomes by BMI in US Adults: The Role of Waist Circumference." *Diabetes/Metabolism Research and Reviews* 33 (5): 1306–12.

Bell, Colin A., L. S. Adair, and B. M. Popkin. 2002. "Ethnic Differences in the Association between Body Mass Index and Hypertension." *American Journal of Epidemiology* 155 (4): 346–53.

de Onis, M., E. Borghi, M. Arimond, P. Webb, T. Croft, K Saha, L. M. De-Regil, F. Thuita, R. Heidkamp, J. Krasevec, C. Hayashi, and R. Flores-Ayala. 2019. "Prevalence Thresholds for Wasting, Overweight and Stunting in Children under 5 Years." *Public Health Nutrition* 22(1): 175–79.

Dietz, W. H. 2017. "Double-Duty Solutions for the Double Burden of Malnutrition." *The Lancet* 390 (10113): 2607–08.

Dinsa, G. D., Y. Goryakin, E. Fumagalli, and M. Suhrcke. 2012. "Obesity and Socioeconomic Status in Developing Countries: A Systematic Review." *Obesity Reviews* 13 (11): 1067–79.

Doak, C., L. Adair, M. Bentley, Z. Fengying, and B. Popkin. 2002. "The Underweight/Overweight Household: An Exploration of Household Sociodemographic and Dietary Factors in China." *Public Health Nutrition* 5 (1A): 215–21.

Doak, C. M., L. S. Adair, M. Bentley, C. Monteiro, and B. M. Popkin. 2005. "The Dual Burden Household and the Nutrition Transition Paradox." *International Journal of Obesity* 29 (1): 129–36.

Doak, C. M., L. S. Adair, C. Monteiro, and B. M. Popkin. 2000. "Overweight and Underweight Coexist within Households in Brazil, China and Russia." *Journal of Nutrition* 130 (12): 2965–71.

Esser, N., S. Legrand-Poels, J. Piette, A. J. Scheen, and N. Paquot. 2014. "Inflammation as a Link between Obesity, Metabolic Syndrome and Type 2 Diabetes." *Diabetes Research and Clinical Practice* 105 (2): 141–50.

Felson, D. T., J. J. Anderson, A. Naimark, A. M. Walker, and R. F. Meenan. 1988. "Obesity and Knee Osteoarthritis: The Framingham Study." *Annals of Internal Medicine* 109 (1): 18–24.

Garrett, J., and M. Ruel. 2005. "Stunted Child–Overweight Mother Pairs: Prevalence and Association with Economic Development and Urbanization." *Food and Nutrition Bulletin* 26 (2): 209–21.

GBD 2015 Obesity Collaborators. 2017. "Health Effects of Overweight and Obesity in 195 Countries over 25 Years." *New England Journal of Medicine* 377 (1): 13–27.

Hardy, L. L., S. Mihrshahi, J. Gale, B. A. Drayton, A. Bauman, and J. Mitchell. 2017. "30-Year Trends in Overweight, Obesity and Waist-to-Height Ratio by Socioeconomic Status in Australian Children, 1985 to 2015." *International Journal of Obesity* 41 (1): 76.

Jaacks, L. M., M. M. Slining, and B. M. Popkin. 2015. "Recent Underweight and Overweight Trends by Rural-Urban Residence among Women in Low- and Middle-Income Countries." *Journal of Nutrition* 145: 352–57.

Jones-Smith, J. C., P. Gordon-Larsen, A. Siddiqi, and B. M. Popkin. 2011. "Cross-National Comparisons of Time Trends in Overweight Inequality by Socioeconomic Status among Women Using Repeated Cross-Sectional Surveys from 37 Developing Countries, 1989–2007." *American Journal of Epidemiology* 173 (6): 667–75.

———. 2012a. "Emerging Disparities in Overweight by Educational Attainment in Chinese Adults (1989–2006)." *International Journal of Obesity* 36 (6): 866–75.

———. 2012b. "Is the Burden of Overweight Shifting to the Poor across the Globe? Time Trends among Women in 39 Low- and Middle-Income Countries (1991–2008)." *International Journal of Obesity* 36 (8): 1114–20.

Joshi, P., S. Islam, P. Pais, S. Reddy, P. Dorairaj, K. Kazmi, M. R. Pandey, S. Haque, S. Mendis, and S. Rangarajan. 2007. "Risk Factors for Early Myocardial Infarction in South Asians Compared with Individuals in Other Countries." *JAMA* 297 (3): 286–94.

Knai, C., T. Lobstein, N. Darmon, H. Rutter, and M. McKee. 2012. "Socioeconomic Patterning of Childhood Overweight Status in Europe." *International Journal of Environmental Research and Public Health* 9 (4): 1472–89.

Kuzawa, C. W., P. C. Hallal, L. Adair, S. K. Bhargava, C. H. Fall, N. Lee, S. A. Norris, C. Osmond, M. Ramirez-Zea, and H. S. Sachdev. 2012. "Birth Weight, Postnatal Weight Gain, and Adult Body Composition in Five Low and Middle Income Countries." *American Journal of Human Biology* 24 (1): 5–13.

Mendez, M. A., C. A. Monteiro, and B. M. Popkin. 2005. "Overweight Exceeds Underweight among Women in Most Developing Countries." *American Journal of Clinical Nutrition* 81 (3): 714–21.

Misra, A. 2015. "Ethnic-Specific Criteria for Classification of Body Mass Index: A Perspective for Asian Indians and American Diabetes Association Position Statement." *Diabetes Technology and Therapeutics* 17 (9): 667–71.

Monteiro, C. A., W. L. Conde, and B. M. Popkin. 2001. "Independent Effects of Income and Education on the Risk of Obesity in the Brazilian Adult Population." *Journal of Nutrition* 131 (3): 881S–6S.

———. 2007. "Income-Specific Trends in Obesity in Brazil: 1975–2003." *American Journal of Public Health* 97 (10): 1808–12.

Monteiro, C. A., M. H. D'A Benicio, W. L. Conde, and B. M. Popkin. 2000. "Shifting Obesity Trends in Brazil." *European Journal of Clinical Nutrition* 54 (4): 342–46.

Nair, M., and D. Prabhakaran. 2012. "Why Do South Asians Have High Risk for CAD?" *Global Heart* 7 (4): 307–14.

NCD-RisC (NCD Risk Factor Collaboration). 2016. "Trends in Adult Body-Mass Index in 200 Countries from 1975 to 2014: A Pooled Analysis of 1698 Population-Based Measurement Studies with 128.9 Million Participants." *The Lancet* 387 (10026): 1377–96.

———. 2019. "Rising Rural Body-Mass Index Is the Main Driver of the Global Obesity Epidemic in Adults." *Nature* 569 (7755): 260–64.

Ng, S. W., and B. M. Popkin. 2012. "Time Use and Physical Activity: A Shift Away from Movement across the Globe." *Obesity Reviews* 13 (8): 659–80.

Patel, S. R., and F. B. Hu. 2008. "Short Sleep Duration and Weight Gain: A Systematic Review." *Obesity* 16 (3): 643–53.

Popkin, B. M. 2004. "The Nutrition Transition: An Overview of World Patterns of Change." *Nutrition Reviews* 62 (7 Pt 2): S140–43.

Popkin, B. M., C. Corvalan, and L. Grummer-Strawn. 2019. "Dynamics of the Double Burden of Malnutrition and the Changing Nutrition Reality." *The Lancet.* https://doi.org/10.1016/S0140-6736(19)32497-3.

Pries, A. M., A. M. Rehman, S. Filteau, N. Sharma, A. Upadhyay, and E. L. Ferguson. 2019. "Unhealthy Snack Food and Beverage Consumption Is Associated with Lower Dietary Adequacy and Length-for-Age z-Scores among 12–23-Month-Olds in Kathmandu Valley, Nepal." *The Journal of Nutrition.* https://doi.org /10.1093/jn/nxz140.

Shrimpton, R., and C. Rokx. 2012. "The Double Burden of Malnutrition: A Review of Global Evidence." Health, Nutrition, and Population Discussion Paper, World Bank, Washington, DC.

Stein, A. D., M. Wang, R. Martorell, S. A. Norris, L. S. Adair, I. Bas, H. S. Sachdev, S. K. Bhargava, C. H. Fall, D. P. Gigante, and C. G. Victora. 2010. "Growth Patterns in Early Childhood and Final Attained Stature: Data from Five Birth Cohorts from Low- and Middle-Income Countries." *American Journal of Human Biology* 22 (3): 353–59.

UNICEF, WHO, and World Bank (United Nations Children's Fund, World Health Organization, and World Bank). 2016. *Joint Child Malnutrition Estimates.* Global Database on Child Growth and Malnutrition. https://www.who.int /nutgrowthdb/estimates2016/en/ (accessed July 2017).

Victora, C. G., L. Adair, C. Fall, P. C. Hallal, R. Martorell, L. Richter, and H. S. Sachdev. 2008. "Maternal and Child Undernutrition: Consequences for Adult Health and Human Capital." *The Lancet* 371 (9609): 340–57.

Watts, A.W., S. M. Mason, K. Loth, N. Larson, and D. Neumark-Sztainer. 2016. "Socioeconomic Differences in Overweight and Weight-Related Behaviors across Adolescence and Young Adulthood: 10-Year Longitudinal Findings from Project EAT." *Preventive Medicine* 87: 194–99.

WCRF and AICR (World Cancer Research Fund and American Institute for Cancer Research). 2018. *Diet, Nutrition, Physical Activity and Cancer: A Global Perspective (A Summary of the Third Expert Report).* Continuous Update Project Expert Report

2018. London: WCRF. https://www.wcrf.org/sites/default/files/Summary-third -expert-report.pdf.

Wells, J. C., E. Pomeroy, S. R. Walimbe, B. M. Popkin, and C. S. Yajnik. 2016. "The Elevated Susceptibility to Diabetes in India: An Evolutionary Perspective." *Frontiers in Public Health* 4: 145.

Wells, J. C., A L. Sawaya, R. Wibeak, M. Mwangome, M. S. Poullas, R. Yajnik, and A. Demaio. Forthcoming. "Emerging Biological Pathways in the Double Burden of Malnutrition." *The Lancet.*

Wells, J. C., R. Wibaek, and M. Poullas. 2018. "The Dual Burden of Malnutrition Increases the Risk of Cesarean Delivery: Evidence From India." *Frontiers in Public Health* 6.

WHO (World Health Organization). 2011. "Haemoglobin Concentrations for the Diagnosis of Anaemia and Assessment of Severity." WHO, Geneva. https:// apps.who.int/iris/handle/10665/85839.

———. 2012. "WHO BMI Classification." http://apps.who.int/bmi/index.jsp ?introPage=intro_3.html.

———. 2017. "The Double Burden of Malnutrition." Policy brief. WHO, Geneva. https://www.who.int/nutrition/publications/doubleburdenmalnutrition -policybrief/en/.

WHO Expert Consultation. 2004. "Appropriate Body-Mass Index for Asian Populations and Its Implications for Policy and Intervention Strategies." *The Lancet* 363 (9403): 157–63.

WHO Multicentre Growth Reference Study Group. 2006. *WHO Child Growth Standards: Length/Height-for-Age, Weight-for-Age, Weight-for-Length, Weight-for-Height and Body Mass Index-for-Age: Methods and Development.* Geneva: WHO. https://www.who.int/childgrowth/standards/Technical_report.pdf?ua=1.

Ziraba, A. K., J. C. Fotso, and R. Ochako. 2009. "Overweight and Obesity in Urban Africa: A Problem of the Rich or the Poor?" *BMC Public Health* 9 (1): 465.

3

Health and Economic Impacts of Overweight/Obesity

Pia Schneider, Barry Popkin, Meera Shekar, Julia Dayton Eberwein, Charlotte Block, and Kyoko Shibata Okamura

Key Messages

- Being overweight/obese puts an individual at higher risk of morbidity and mortality from non-communicable diseases (NCDs): the heavier the person and the longer the person has carried excess weight, the higher the risks.
- Overweight/obesity-related NCDs are among the top-three killers in every region of the world except Sub-Saharan Africa. Childhood overweight/obesity is particularly damaging. It puts the child at high risk of developing debilitating NCDs and living with them longer, denying the child her or his full health and economic potential.
- Low- and middle-income country contexts, which include weak health care systems already burdened with high prevalence of infectious disease, create additional challenges to preventing and treating the health consequences of overweight and obesity.
- Overweight/obesity reduces productivity and increases absenteeism, disability rates, and the risk of earlier retirement.
- The estimated economic costs of overweight/obesity vary considerably since studies use different methodologies to estimate direct and indirect costs.

- The shift in diets and activity patterns linked to increased overweight/obesity are also linked to important water and carbon emissions concerns, thus perpetuating what is termed by the *Lancet* Commission on Obesity (LCO) as the *syndemic of undernutrition, obesity, and climate change*. That report also highlights potential double- and triple-duty actions that will provide climate co-benefits in addition to addressing overweight/obesity and undernutrition. The *Lancet* EAT Commission report also advocates a shift toward more sustainable plant-based diets to address both overweight/obesity and climate change.
- Whatever estimates of costs one might subscribe to, the big picture message is that growing health care costs linked to increasing overweight/obesity rates are a trend across both the developed and developing world. And there are climate co-benefits to changing food systems to promote healthier diets. Prevention of overweight/obesity therefore makes sense from a public finance perspective. Governments have a key role to play in this effort, including by ensuring that consumers are informed about their health and the consequences of their dietary and lifestyle choices.

The Health Impact: Why Overweight/Obesity Matters

Overweight/obesity by itself puts an individual at greater risk for mortality, but it is also part of a progressive disease state that starts with carrying excessive weight and leads to the development of NCDs such as type 2 diabetes, cardiovascular disease, and cancers (figure 3.1, box 3.1). An extensive description of all the cancers linked to overweight/obesity is found elsewhere (WCRF and AICR 2018). Overweight/obesity is increasingly seen as a major preventable cause for cancers, diabetes, and other NCDs.

Table 3.1 presents the overweight/obesity-related risk of developing NCDs. In general, the heavier a person is and the longer he or she is overweight/obese, the higher the risk of developing and dying from NCDs (Abdullah 2015; Martin-Rodriguez et al. 2015; WCRF and AICR 2018). For example, an overweight man is over twice as likely as a man with a healthy weight to develop diabetes; an overweight woman has an almost four times greater risk. The risk increases greatly if the individual is obese: obese men are almost seven times more likely and women over 12 times more likely to have diabetes than normal-weight adults. Excess weight confers a much greater risk for women than men of developing some NCDs, including kidney cancer, hypertension, and coronary artery disease. Men are at higher risk for pancreatic cancer and osteoarthritis (Guh et al. 2009).

Figure 3.1 Health Impacts of Overweight/Obesity

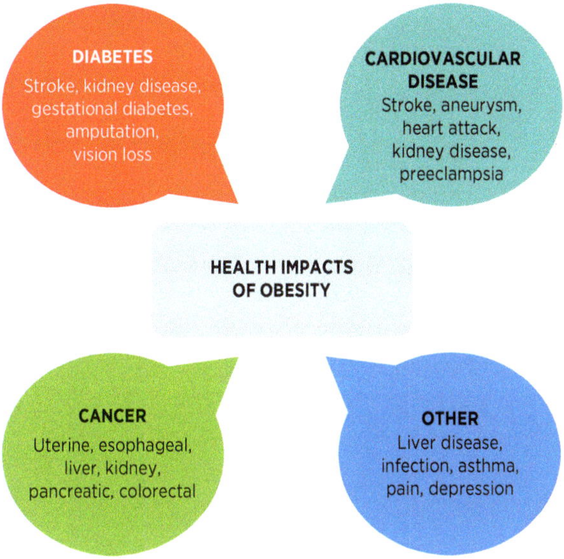

DIABETES
Stroke, kidney disease, gestational diabetes, amputation, vision loss

CARDIOVASCULAR DISEASE
Stroke, aneurysm, heart attack, kidney disease, preeclampsia

HEALTH IMPACTS OF OBESITY

CANCER
Uterine, esophageal, liver, kidney, pancreatic, colorectal

OTHER
Liver disease, infection, asthma, pain, depression

BOX 3.1

Obesity: Both a Disease and a Risk Factor

Obesity is a complex condition. It has long been considered a risk factor for other diseases, especially non-communicable diseases (NCDs, as described in this chapter). Debate has centered on whether all cases of obesity should be categorized in the same way, because obesity can exist with and without comorbidities and therefore treatment requirements vary. Within the past several decades, more and more medical and health entities—such as the World Health Organization, the Asia Oceania Association for the Study of Obesity, and the American Medical Association—have declared obesity to be a disease state. Obese individuals without comorbidities are still at risk for developing the *disease of obesity*—a condition by which obesity is accompanied by additional comorbidities such as high blood pressure, high blood glucose, or high cholesterol. Obesity by itself increases risk of mortality, and obesity disease, with obesity-related NCDs, puts an obese individual at greater risk for morbidity and mortality (Bray et al. 2017; Kyle, Dhurandhar, and Allison 2016; Lobstein et al. 2017).

Table 3.1   Body Fatness and Risk of Cancer Incidence: Evidence from the WCRF/AICR Third Expert Report

Cancer site	Exposure and increment (measure of body fatness)	Risk estimates (relative risk) number of studies; number of cases		
		Overall	Men	Women
WCRF/AICR conclusion:[a] *Convincing: Increases risk*				
Oesophagus (adenocarcinoma)	BMI per 5 kg/m²	1.48 (1.35–1.62) studies = 9; cases =1,725	1.56 (1.39–1.74) studies = 3; cases = NR	1.48 (1.29–1.71) studies = 3; cases = NR
Pancreas	BMI per 5 kg/m²	1.10 (1.07–1.14) studies = 23; cases = 9,504	1.13 (1.04–1.22) studies = NR; cases = NR	1.10 (1.04–1.16) studies = NR; cases = NR
Liver	BMI per 5 kg/m²	1.30 (1.16–1.46) studies = 12; cases = 14,311	1.21 (1.02–1.44) studies = 8; cases = NR	1.21 (1.10–1.33) studies = 4; cases = NR
Colorectum	BMI per 5 kg/m²	1.05 (1.03–1.07) studies = 38; cases = 71,089	1.08 (1.04–1.11) studies = 20; cases = NR	1.05 (1.02–1.08) studies = 24; cases = NR
Breast (postmenopause)	BMI per 5 kg/m²	n.a.	n.a.	1.12 (1.09–1.15) studies = 56; cases = 80,404
Endometrium	BMI per 5 kg/m²	n.a.	n.a.	1.50 (1.42–1.59) studies = 26; cases = 18,717
Kidney	BMI per 5 kg/m²	1.30 (1.25–1.35) studies = 23; cases = 15,575	1.29 (1.23–1.36) studies = NR; cases = NR	1.28 (1.24–1.32) studies = NR; cases = NR

continued next page

Table 3.1 *(continued)*

Cancer site	Exposure and increment (measure of body fatness)	Risk estimates (relative risk) number of studies; number of cases		
		Overall	Men	Women
WCRF/AICR conclusion:[a] *Probable: Increases risk*				
Mouth, pharynx, and larynx	BMI per 5 kg/m^2	1.15 (1.06–1.24) studies = 20; cases = 796	*	*
Stomach (cardia)	BMI per 5 kg/m^2	1.23 (1.07–1.40) studies = 7; cases = 2,050	1.13 (0.98–1.30) studies = 3; cases = 360	*
Gallbladder	BMI per 5 kg/m^2	1.25 (1.15–1.37) studies = 8; cases = 6,004		
Ovary	BMI per 5 kg/m^2	n.a.		
Prostate (advanced)	BMI per 5 kg/m^2	n.a.		
WCRF/AICR conclusion:[a] *Limited – suggestive: Increases risk*				
Cervix[b]	BMI per 5 kg/m^2	n.a.	n.a.	1.02 (0.97–1.07) studies = 9; cases = 5,144

Source: WCRF and AICR 2018. Available at dietandcancerreport.org. Reproduced with permission.

Note: This table is based on a Cochrane style meta-analysis conducted by a global panel of scholars with WCRF staff assisting. BMI = body mass index; n.a. = not applicable; NR = not reported; WCRF/AICR = World Cancer Research Fund/American Institute for Cancer Research.

a. For a full description of the definitions of, and the criteria for, the terminology of *convincing, probable,* and *limited – suggestive* please see *Judging the Evidence* (WCRF and AICR 2018), available at wcrf.org/dietandcancer/judging-the-evidence.

b. There is no evidence of effect modification by menopausal status for body fatness and the risk of endometrial, ovarian, or cervical cancer so the evidence of all women (irrespective of menopausal status) is presented together.

* Not possible to conduct analysis stratified by sex.

It is important to note that these relative risks and the related disability-adjusted life years (DALYs) are based on epidemiological studies and assumptions that mainly include non-Hispanic white populations from the United States, the United Kingdom, and other high-income countries (Albrecht, Mayer-Davis, and Popkin 2017; Bell, Adair, and Popkin 2002; WHO Expert Consultation 2004; WHO Western Pacific Region 2000).[1] These risks ignore to a great extent the increased risk of hypertension, diabetes, heart disease, and cancers that can be linked to body-mass index (BMI) levels below 25 in low- and middle-income countries (WHO Expert Consultation 2004), as noted in chapter 2. Because these estimates are based on limited population groups, the real costs in terms of DALYs lost will be much greater.

The Global Burden of Disease study estimates that overweight/obesity-related disease causes about 4 million deaths a year, or about 7 percent of deaths from all causes (GBD 2015 Obesity Collaborators 2017). Overweight/obesity also contributes approximately 120 million DALYs, or about 5 percent of DALYs from all causes. Among many other overweight/obesity-related illnesses, cardiovascular disease is the first major contributor of deaths and DALYs, followed by type 2 diabetes (second contributor of deaths) and chronic kidney disease (second contributor of DALYs). Large increases in attributable DALYs between 1990 and 2016 have been seen among the 20 illnesses for which there is evidence of association with high BMI. Type 2 diabetes and osteoarthritis have had the largest increase in DALYs, doubling their impact over the last decades (GBD 2015 Obesity Collaborators 2017).

Multiple factors influence the health impact of overweight/obesity. First is the relatively unknown area of genetics, which is not amenable to action. Second is the long-term impact of stunting and malnutrition during the first 1,000 days of life; this may also be the reason why the influence of lower BMI levels is larger on many low- and middle-income-country populations than in non-Hispanic white populations. Stunting in the first 1,000 days appears to affect visceral fat (central adiposity) more than overall overweight/obesity and also the health consequences of visceral fat. The third are dietary causes.

The second of these factors may be less obvious. Major shifts in the prevalence of stunting have occurred over the past four decades in low- and middle-income countries. However, it is important to note that there is a considerable lag between stunting during the preschool period and the subsequent increased risk of becoming overweight/obese with all its related complications (Wells, Wibaek, and Poullas 2018). This proposition of the links between low birthweights and adult chronic diseases was first proposed as the Barker Hypothesis (Barker 1990; Law et al. 1992); subsequent research has refined this understanding, so now the focus is on fetal and infant development that is linked to reduced height (stunting) as the major measurable pathway. The literature suggests that stunting is more closely associated with increased risks of an array of NCDs and some increased risks of overweight/obesity, particularly in the most critical visceral fat measures (Adair et al. 2013; Kuzawa et al. 2011). The levels of stunting seen in the 1990s, for example, will be reflected now, in 2019, only by those in the 20-to-30-year-old age group. This lag indicates that many low- and middle-income countries will see future rises in overweight/obesity linked both to the high stunting rates and to the reduced energy expenditure and changing food patterns discussed in the next chapter (Adair et al. 2013; Stein et al. 2010; Victora et al. 2008).

The Economic Costs of Overweight/Obesity

Overweight/obesity creates a need for health care to treat higher incidence of chronic diseases such as diabetes and heart disease. It can lead to disability and earlier retirement, and can also lower productivity. Chronic diseases require medical treatment that contributes to higher health expenditures.

Several studies have attempted to estimate the economic costs of overweight/obesity. However, each study uses different methodologies and differing definitions of direct and indirect costs of overweight/obesity, making comparison difficult.

An unpublished systematic review of published studies conducted for this report (by Ana Perez Exposito) identified 34 studies between 2007 and 2017 that estimated the national costs of overweight, obesity, or both. These 34 studies cover 13 countries, 3 of which are middle-income countries (Brazil, China, and Thailand) and 10 are high-income countries. No lower-income countries were included in these studies. The results suggest an estimated cost range (share of GDP lost) of 0.01 percent in Brazil to 2.08 percent in the United States for both obesity and overweight (18 studies), and 0.00 percent (Brazil) to 4.78 percent in the United States for obesity only. In the United States these costs are estimated to be between US$300 and more than US$3,000 per capita (between US$89 billion and US$212 billion in total costs); estimates in other high-income countries are much lower. Another estimate from the United States suggests that overweight/obesity costs the government, employers, and individuals about US$147 billion per year; however, this cost will rise significantly as medical treatment for chronic diseases becomes more sophisticated. One estimate from Indonesia (Kosen 2018) suggests losses of about 3 percent of GDP, equivalent to about US$28.4 billion; another global estimate suggests losses of 2.8 percent of GDP, equal to about US$2.0 trillion (Dobbs et al. 2014).

A recently published systematic review (Tremmel et al. 2017) lays out the methodological challenges of comparing the results from these studies. Table 3.2 summarizes some of the recent estimates, which demonstrate a variety of definitions applied for "direct" and "indirect" costs. Within these categories, different types of costs are measured—for example, the health care costs incurred by a person that stem from overweight/obesity as well as the obesity-related treatment costs incurred by the health system. These differences are relevant to projections about possible savings if the prevalence of obesity were to be reduced.

A summary of estimated costs of overweight/obesity from various countries (Qin and Pan 2016) is presented in table 3.3.

These estimates also reiterate a wide range of costs associated with overweight/obesity—between US$300 to more than US$3,000 per capita in the United States (between US$89 billion and US$212 billion in total costs), versus much lower estimates in other high-income countries. Combined with the fact that overweight/obesity rates in the United States are on the rise and life expectancy is declining (especially as compared with countries such as France, Germany, Japan, and the United Kingdom), this should be a cause for major concern among policy makers. In Germany, the direct costs were estimated at €8,647 million, corresponding to 3.27 percent of total German health care expenditures in 2008, with additional indirect costs of €8,150 million, of which two-thirds were costs of workdays lost.

In China, the estimates of health care costs associated with overweight/obesity rose from 3.13 percent of China's annual national health care expenditure in 2009 to 0.56 percent in 2000. In Brazil, overweight/obesity-related health care costs are expected to double from US$5.8 billion in 2010 to US$10.1 billion in 2050. All of this shows that increasing health care costs linked to increasing overweight/obesity rates are a trend across the world.

The Economic Factors That Affect Overweight/Obesity

Two major sets of theories relate to the economic causes of overweight/obesity. One connects it to the major shifts in technology and hence reduced activity; the other relates to the relative price of food—the price of healthy and unhealthy foods and the way these prices focus consumption on lower-priced ultra-processed foods, refined starchy staples, and a high-calorie diet relative to energy expenditure (Cutler, Glaeser, and Shapiro 2003; Finkelstein et al. 2008; Finkelstein and Strombotne 2010). Most of the literature focuses on high-income countries. Few longitudinal rigorous analyses from lower-income countries exist, but one long-term study has shown that declining physical activity played a major role—which in turn

Table 3.2 The Economic Costs of Overweight/Obesity

Country/region and year	Characteristics	Study	Methodology	Estimated costs
International (Australia, Canada, Finland, Germany, Republic of Korea, Netherlands, New Zealand, Sweden, and the United States) 2017	Estimated indirect costs International comparison Not a meta-analysis (graphical comparison)	Goettler, Grosse, and Sonntag 2017	*Indirect costs* defined as the losses from reduced work productivity due to short-term and long-term inability to work, including "temporary work loss" such as sick leave ("absenteeism") and reduced productivity while being present at work ("presenteeism"), permanent work loss such as disability pension and premature death.	Because of the methodological heterogeneity, no aggregated/comparative figures were proposed.
United States 2018	Estimated direct and indirect costs	Waters and Graf 2018	*Direct costs* calculated from the Medical Expenditure Panel Survey (including household survey and insurance data), using the concept of the treated prevalence of health conditions that are associated with obesity in overweight/obese adults, compared to normal weight individuals. Methodology/definition of *indirect costs* is not mentioned.	In 2016, the cost of chronic diseases attributable to the prevalence of obesity and overweight resulted in a US$1.72 trillion price tag, equivalent to 9.3% of US GDP (US$480.7 billion in direct health care costs and US$1.24 trillion in indirect costs due to lost economic productivity). This makes up 47.1% of the total cost of chronic diseases nationwide.
Republic of Ireland; Northern Ireland 2015	Estimated direct and indirect costs	Dee et al. 2015	Included *direct costs* as health care utilization costs and drug costs and *indirect costs* as work absenteeism and premature mortality.	Republic of Ireland: In 2009 €437 million in direct costs (health care costs) and €865 million in indirect costs (productivity loss due to overweight/obesity). Northern Ireland: In 2009, €127.41 million in direct costs (health care costs) and €362 million in indirect costs (productivity loss).

continued next page

Table 3.2 (*continued*)

Country/region and year	Characteristics	Study	Methodology	Estimated costs
Germany 2015	Estimated direct and indirect costs Estimated the increase in the costs between two time points (2002 and 2008) by updating the 2002 research	Lehnert et al. 2015	*Direct costs* estimated for inpatient/outpatient treatment, rehabilitation, and *other direct costs* (including health protection, ambulance, administration, research and evaluation, investments, and other facilities). *Indirect costs* calculated as loss of productivity from paid and unpaid work due to sickness absence, early retirement, and mortality, applying the human capital approach.	Total costs attributable to excess weight (BMI > 25kg/m²) in Germany in 2008 amounted to €16,797 million (up 70% compared to 2002). Direct costs were €8,647 million, corresponding to 3.27% of total German heath care expenditures in 2008. Indirect costs were €8,150 million in 2008 (up 62% compared to 2002), of which two-thirds (€5,276 million) were costs of unpaid work (up 75% compared to 2002).
China 2016	Estimated direct costs Per capita and share of national health care expenditure Uses longitudinal data from 2000–2009 China Health and Nutrition Surveys	Qin and Pan 2016	*Direct costs* based on medical expenditures calculated using the China Health and Nutrition Survey (2002, 2004, 2006, 2009), which includes self-medication expenses (for example, over-the-counter drugs) and formal health costs (impatient, outpatient, preventive services) including both insurance providers' and out-of-pocket payments.	The per capita medical cost attributable to obesity and overweight in a single medical event is estimated to be 6.18 yuan, or 5.29% of the total personal medical expenditure. This translates to 24.35 billion yuan annual cost on the national scale, accounting for 2.46% of China's national health care expenditure. The subsample analyses also show that costs are higher for urban dwellers, women, and for the better educated, and it increases over time.

continued next page

Table 3.2 *(continued)*

Country/region and year	Characteristics	Study	Methodology	Estimated costs
Republic of Korea 2018	Estimated direct costs Estimated the cost over 11 years, using the longitudinal database	Song et al. 2018	*Direct costs* were calculated using the National Health Insurance Service–Health Screening Cohort data that includes insurance eligibility, medical treatments, medical care institutions, and general examinations. Overweight (BMI 23–24.99) and obesity I (25–29.99), II (30–34.99), and III (35–59.99) were defined by Asian BMI criteria.	Obese individuals with BMI ≥ 30 had medical expenditures of 1.21–1.40 times those of normal weight individuals over approximately 11 years (after being adjusted for age, sex, income level, and comorbidities)
Brazil 2013	Estimated direct costs	Rtveladze et al. 2013	The study projects an increase in health care costs of obesity-related diseases between two time points (2010 and 2050), but the estimates are not derived from comparison between overweight/obese and normal-weight counterparts.	Health care costs will double from 2010 (US$5.8 billion) in 2050 alone (US$10.1 billion). Over 40 years costs will reach US$330 billion, based on the model that projects an increase in the overweight/obesity prevalence in Brazilian male population from 57% in 2010 to 95% by 2050.

Source: Original compilation (see the References section of the chapter for full study information).

Note: BMI = body mass index.

Table 3.3 Summary of Estimated Costs of Overweight/Obesity in Selected Countries

Country	Study	Cost (2010 US$, millions)	Percentage of national medical costs	Per capita cost (2010 US$)
Australia	Access Economics 2006	675.30	1.3	32.41
Canada	Katzmarzyk and Janssen 2004	1,577.90	2.2	48.54
France	Emery et al. 2007	2,368.00–7,126.00	1.5–4.6	90.25
Germany	Konnopka, Bödemann, and König 2011	5,579.00	2.1	67.82
Korea, Rep.	Kang et al. 2011	1,787.00	3.7	36.56
Spain	Vazquez-Sanchez and Lam 2002	1,001.00	1.7	22.25
Sweden	Swedish Council on Technology Assessment in Health Care 2002	182.62–365.34	1.0–2.0	30.00
United Kingdom	House of Commons Health Select Committee 2004	1,790.00–2,000.00	2.3–2.6	32.22
United States	Finkelstein, Fiebelkorn, and Wang 2003	89,415.10	5.7	302.35
United States	Finkelstein et al. 2009	148,902.80	10.0	503.50
United States	Cawley and Meyerhoefer 2012	212,462.00	20.6	3,059.00

Source: Based on Qin and Pan 2016.

links to the technology issue (Ng et al. 2012). More recently, economists point to the relatively higher costs of healthy food globally. As noted in chapter 2, it is this balance between energy expenditure and the metabolic effects of various types of food that jointly affects weight gain.

Economic theory assumes that perfectly informed consumers will maximize their utility by consuming various goods depending on their relative prices as well as on the consumers' income and preferences. This means that changes in prices and income influence how much of different goods rational consumers will buy, as will their preferences for different products.

Relative Price

The price of a good is inversely related to the demand for it. According to consumer theory, if prices decrease, demand will go up. Over the past decades, prices for food and beverages have increased globally—but not all prices have increased equally. Some products saw a higher price increase than others, which resulted in a change in the relative price across products. For example, U.S. data point to substantial differences in price increases across products in the past 35 years. Prices for fresh fruits and vegetables rose by 190 percent, compared with a 66 percent increase for sweets and sugar. Low-income households are particularly wary about food prices because food makes up a large share of their household consumption basket (Drewnowski and Specter 2004). They are therefore most likely to adjust their consumption and shift from higher-priced items to cheaper products even though these substitutes may be less healthy and higher in calories and sugar, which contributes to weight gains (Epstein et al. 2012).

In general, across the developing world, it is the relative reduced price of unhealthy ultra-processed food along with their ingredients—such as refined flours, sugars, and edible oils—that have fueled a major shift in global food intake toward less healthy foods. In addition to the shift in global relative and absolute prices for these highly processed foods and beverages compared with prices for healthier legumes, vegetables, and fruits, among other items, there has been a long-term global decline in the price of animal-source foods, particularly beef (Popkin 2011). The change in beef prices led the International Food Policy Research Institute (IFPRI) and others to speak about a "beef revolution" (discussed as a major increase in global beef consumption as the driver of animal-source food consumption trends) (Delgado 2003; Delgado et al. 1999). However, from more recent trends, this appears to have shifted to the current "poultry revolution" whereby much of the more recent increase in animal-source food consumption has come from poultry globally (see Zhai et al. [2014] for an example from China). But again, as a vast array of research on price elasticity, food taxation, and related topics has shown, it is the relative price of various healthy versus unhealthy foods and beverages that matters (Deaton and Muellbauer 1980; Timmer and Alderman 1979). Lower prices for sugary beverages and ultra-processed foods is one of the arguments for governments to tax unhealthy products.

Income and Preferences

A combination of increased income, increased marketing of ultra-processed foods and beverages, and the growth of global media has led to major shifts in food preferences toward much less healthful ultra-processed foods in general and animal-source foods in low- and middle-income countries

(Chaudri and Timmer 1986; Monteiro et al. 2013; Popkin 2008, 2014; Popkin and Reardon 2018). Concurrent rapid penetration by modern retailers has also been linked to these shifts, particularly in low-income areas where retailers selling fresh products are not readily available (Popkin and Reardon 2018).

The result of these combined factors has been a marked increase in the demand for both ultra-processed foods and animal-source foods. Worldwide, the demand for food and beverages has increased, as shown by higher total calorie intake per capita. The World Health Organization (WHO) estimates that average daily per capita food consumption in the developing world has increased by 400 kilocalories: from 2,405 kilocalories per capita per day in 1985 to 2,850 in 2015.[2] To some extent, higher demand is driven by more income as well as by the retail revolution, increased food marketing, and reduced prices for ultra-processed foods (Reardon et al. 2003; Tschirley et al. 2015). In addition, food consumption patterns tend to change as per capita incomes rise (see chapter 2). Low-income households are more susceptible to price changes and will consume fewer fruits and vegetables and less fiber, but more fat and sugar-sweetened beverages than the better-off (Drewnowski and Specter 2004).

Preferences have changed too, as more diverse products become available. Much of the increase in calories in consumption is caused by the increased availability of high-caloric ready-to-eat and ready-to-heat snack food and beverages as well as energy-dense and nutrient-poor food prepared by the formal and informal retail and food service sectors. Critical regional patterns to these changes as well as unique factors in each country exist; nevertheless, snacking on convenience foods (an activity that in the nineteenth century did not exist) has been a major part of the increased caloric intake in both high-income countries and low- and middle-income countries in the past 40 years. How to differentiate the impact of modern marketing and affluence on these snacking behaviors is unclear. Countries as diverse as Brazil, Mexico, and the United States are among those where over a fifth of kilocalories are coming from snacks, and there is evidence of an explosion in snacking in China (Duffey, Pereira, and Popkin 2013; Duffey, Rivera, and Popkin 2014; Dunford and Popkin 2017; Erlanson-Albertsson and Zetterstrom 2005; Huffman et al. 2014; Popkin 2008; Roester 2017; Seabrook 2011; Wang et al. 2012) as well as most recently in Nepal (Pries et al. 2019).

Modern Technologies, Energy Expenditure, and Lifestyle Changes

A combination of globalization, trade agreements, and the push to find cheaper labor markets along with most development initiatives has led to the introduction of an array of modern technologies that affect energy expenditure at work and lifestyles in both urban and rural areas (for example, the introduction of computers, small gas-driven cheap plows, modern irrigation pumps, and electricity in rural areas; see Herrin 1979). Moreover, this push has affected home-based work (with refrigeration, rice cookers, water piped into houses and villages, and propane stoves), transportation (with motorized vehicles of all sorts), and leisure (with the arrival of television and smart phones), and how much time people spend "moving." These effects demonstrate that many technologies have led to enormous declines in energy expenditure in the past four decades in low- and middle-income countries (Ng, Norton, and Popkin 2009; Ng and Popkin 2012). It is important to note that they come at a time when, based on the WHO data cited above, caloric intake appears to be increasing.

As a result, lifestyles have become much more sedentary and people now expend fewer calories since they are working in jobs that require less physical activity. This means that people will also need fewer calories than they expend. Individuals with higher incomes will have more opportunities to offset increased calorie consumption through physical activity, for example, by joining a gym. However, for lower-income households, this may not be an option as they may not be able to afford high membership fees; they may reside in densely populated urban areas where walking or jogging is difficult and personal safety is often a great concern. They may also incur opportunity costs for their time if they have to work longer hours to make ends meet (Drewnowski and Specter 2004).

Expectation of Health Effect

In addition to consumption theory, economic theory also uses expected utility theory to explain how uncertainty affects individuals' decisions and behavior. Using expected utility theory, it can be argued that individuals make choices between an uncertain "health loss" due to obesity that may likely occur in the future and a certain financial loss caused by paying a higher price for fruits and vegetables today to prevent obesity. This uncertainty about an expected future outcome affects their behavior today. Expected utility theory assumes that people are risk averse. They make choices about what risk to take as it has implications for their overall wealth, which includes their health status. If individuals are rational, they will go for certainty and pay a higher price today for healthy products to prevent a future loss (illness related to overweight). However, through modern medicine, people can level out different risks over time, and this affects their choices about how to behave. They will pay less today for unhealthy food knowing they are taking a health risk (weight gain). But this risk and its consequences become less risky through modern medicine and medical coverage.

Access to modern medicine therefore alleviates the health consequences of being overweight or obese for individuals. This is especially the case where government and health insurance pay for care and individual out-of-pocket payment is low. It could therefore be argued that individuals are less inclined to pay a higher price for healthy food today to prevent obesity, because they do not think about future health problems as much as current costs or they know they will have access to relatively inexpensive health care in case they need it in the future. As a result, they will care less about their growing waistline and obesity prevention although they are aware of the possible negative effect on their health status. The resulting impact on government health expenditures is a main argument for governments to invest in prevention and inform people about the negative health consequences of obesity. While such health care is available in Latin America and selected other low- and middle-income countries, it is available in the majority of high-income countries.

The Role of Government

From an economic perspective, obesity becomes a public policy concern if it leads to higher health care costs and market failure and if it threatens equity objectives. These concerns would be reason for government to intervene.

Health Expenditures

As shown in the previous sections, overweight/obesity affects health status and it creates a need for medical care to treat related health consequences. It has been associated with higher incidence of chronic diseases, such as diabetes and heart disease; earlier risk of disability and retirement; and lower life expectancy for some population groups. Chronic diseases require medical treatment that contribute to higher health expenditures. It could be expected that if obesity leads to shorter lifespans, then total health expenditures may be lower for the obese than the non-obese—as, for example, is the case for tobacco consumption. However, findings from the United States suggest that obesity costs the government, employers, and individuals about US$147 billion per year as medical treatment for chronic diseases becomes more sophisticated. Another estimate suggests costs between US$89 billion and US$212 billion in the United States. In China, one estimate that looked at the total costs of overweight and obesity, including the indirect costs of overweight/obesity and related dietary and physical activity patterns, ranged between

3.58 percent and 8.73 percent of gross national product in 2000 and 2025, respectively (Popkin et al. 2006). The estimates of health care costs associated with overweight and obesity rose from 3.13 percent of China's annual national health care expenditure in 2009 to 0.56 percent in 2000 (Qin and Pan 2016). In Brazil, obesity-related health care costs are expected to double from US$5.8 billion in 2010 to US$10.1 billion in 2050 (Rtveladze et al. 2013). Government interventions to prevent overweight/obesity and its health consequences therefore make sense from a public finance perspective, which aims for efficient allocations of funds.

Market Failure

From an economic perspective, overweight/obesity becomes a concern if it leads to market failure; this would be another reason for government to intervene (Begg, Fischer, and Dornbusch 2000). Market failure means that resource allocation through the private sector is not efficient. Market failure can be triggered by (1) externalities, (2) asymmetric information, (3) market power, and (4) public goods characteristics (Finkelstein and Strombotne 2010).

Externality is a reason for government to intervene, but overweight/obesity does not create externalities or negative side-effects on others in the way smoking does on nonsmokers. Although some "quasi-externalities" on individual behavior exist when people live and work in an environment with a higher prevalence of overweight/obese individuals, which may have a self-enforcing effect on unhealthy eating behavior for the group, this increased prevalence does not create any negative impact on others. In addition, excessive medical care costs for treating overweight/obesity may increase insurance costs for normal weight individuals.

Asymmetric or imperfect information is a problem in food consumption because producers know more about the nutrient-content than consumers do and use marketing that is often deceptive to incorrectly inform consumers. To improve information, governments have launched awareness campaigns about what makes up a healthy diet and requested producers to label food packages to inform consumers about content and nutrient value; however, the costs and successes of such campaigns are limited because of extensive marketing of ultra-processed foods and beverages.

Market power means that a single firm or a few firms dominate the market. Because of their market power, firms can dictate the price at which a product is offered, which leads to price increases. Government antitrust agencies are tasked with preventing firms from dictating prices. Price increases are problematic for overweight/obesity because unhealthy food tends to be cheaper, which has led governments to introduce diet-related taxes on these products.

Finally, *public goods* are goods that would not be produced by the private sector—for example, certain health services such as emergency care. However, it would be difficult to argue that overweight/obesity rates are triggered by a shortage of public goods such as health care.

From an economic perspective, therefore, government's role is to intervene and correct for market failure in the private sector. Governments can ensure that consumers are informed about the health consequences of their dietary choices and governments can correct for large differences in relative prices between healthy and unhealthy products and work to limit marketing that increases sales of ultra-processed foods.

Equity in Health

In addition to their role in preventing overweight/obesity to manage health expenditures and correct for asymmetric information, governments intervene to meet equity objectives. Governments may argue for targeted prevention programs for lower-income groups if they and other disadvantaged individuals are more affected by overweight/obesity and do not have the same access to medical treatment for related diseases. Brazil, for example, has issued guidelines to improve equity in access to healthy food, particularly in low-income areas and in schools. In this case, government interventions help ensure that disadvantaged groups are not excluded from good health. Adequate diagnosis and treatment are major issues for the poor in most countries of the world (Gordon-Larsen et al. 2017).

Equity issues represent a major argument for the use of government interventions to prevent obesity. It is often argued that most sin or ultra-processed food and beverage taxes are regressive because the poor spend a higher proportion of their income on goods subject to these taxes than the rich. However, while such indirect taxes reduce the redistribution effect from the rich to the poor, they may still have a pro-poor effect if tax revenues are used by government to finance pro-poor public services such as health care in the public sector that is predominantly used by the poor (Begg, Fischer, and Dornbusch 2000) or if the impact of these taxes improves significantly the health of the poor and prevents overweight/obesity and many NCDs that would otherwise be undiagnosed or poorly treated.

Some population groups, such as children, will need additional protection as they are too young to fully understand the health consequences of consuming unhealthy food and beverages, including alcohol. This has caused governments to focus even more strongly on child health and prevention. In South Africa, the Advertising Standards Authority (ASA) prohibits misleading food marketing and advertising tactics via any form of media, including enticing children with toys and using celebrities and cartoon characters to advertise unhealthy food products to children.

Children's rights are written into constitutions in many low- and middle-income countries. These constitutional rights are used for legal and government challenges to the marketing of ultra-processed foods.

This discussion shows that, from an economic perspective, overweight/obesity is affected by market factors such as relative prices, income, preferences, and technological advances at work and in medicine. Government interventions should therefore focus on overweight/obesity prevention by facilitating information and access and by reducing the relative cost for healthy diets and physical activity, particularly for low-income groups. This would require a comprehensive approach to policy formulation including in agriculture, environment, transport, taxation, and health care.

The Cost of Overweight/Obesity for Climate Co-Benefits and Water Use

Costs of overweight/obesity are linked not only with the outcomes noted above but also with the food and activity dynamics that are linked to global weight increases. The latter ones also have significant impacts on climate with all the related costs (Springmann et al. 2018). The underlying causes of obesity are very much linked to increased water use and carbon emissions. This is true for both the reduced energy expenditures for home and market production and transportation as well as for shifts in dietary patterns. For the food sector, much of the attention has centered on the growing global demand for animal-source food, in particular ruminant animals, whereas the huge growth in the packaged processed food sector has been generally ignored except for a few very focused studies. Both sets of causes are deeply linked to an increased use of energy, increased carbon emissions, and, for food, increased water use.

The current literature suggests that just a shift in global diets to reduced animal-source foods use would not only reduce overweight/obesity but also address much of the global climate problem (EAT *Lancet* Commission 2019; Godfray et al. 2018; Springmann et al. 2018). A major reduction in the production of animal-source foods is one central element that could significantly reduce greenhouse gases. Much of this reduction would come from the reduction in methane emissions from ruminant animals (cows and lambs, in particular). The Food and Agriculture Organization of the United Nations, for example, states that one-third of total emissions from global livestock are related to these animals (FAO 2007). The *Lancet* EAT Commission group showed that their proposed dietary shifts away from ruminant animal-based diets (that is, diets based on beef and lamb) would meet the Paris Accord climate goals (EAT *Lancet* Commission 2019; Springmann et al. 2018).

A healthy diet with fewer sweetened, sugary beverages would also reduce water use because crops that provide the sugar require a great deal of water (Springmann et al. 2018). There is a small literature on water use and sugary beverage intake, but to date no major studies have been published on other aspects of any dimension of climate change related to the production and distribution of the least healthy ultra-processed foods and beverages. This represents a critical gap because there are also major environmental (particularly water and carbon emissions) costs associated with the production of sugary drinks. For a half liter (500 milliliters or 17 ounces) of a regular soft drink, the total water life cycle costs range from 168 liters when the sweetener is derived from sugar beets to 309 liters for sugarcane in India (Ercin, Aldaya, and Hoekstra 2011; Hoekstra 2013; Hoekstra and Chapagain 2007). A major knowledge gap is found in the water and carbon emissions footprint for all other unhealthy ultra-processed foods, which institutions such as the World Bank could help fill in.

Notes

1. DALYs are calculated by summing years of life lost and years of life lived with disability due to each illness.
2. These data are available at the World Health Organization's "Global and Regional Food Consumption Patterns and Trends" at https://www.who.int /nutrition/topics/3_foodconsumption/en/.

References

Abdullah, A. 2015. "The Double Burden of Undernutrition and Overnutrition in Developing Countries: An Update." *Current Obesity Reports* 4 (3): 337–49.

Access Economics. 2006. "The Economic Costs of Obesity: A Report Prepared for Diabetes Australia." http://www.accesseconomics.com.au.

Adair, L. S., C. H. Fall, C. Osmond, A. D. Stein, R. Martorell, M. Ramirez-Zea, H. S. Sachdev, D. L. Dahly, I. Bas, S. A. Norris, L. Micklesfield, P. Hallal, and C. G. Victora. 2013. "Associations of Linear Growth and Relative Weight Gain during Early Life with Adult Health and Human Capital in Countries of Low and Middle Income: Findings from Five Birth Cohort Studies." *The Lancet* 382 (9891): 525–34.

Albrecht, S. S., E. Mayer-Davis, and B. M. Popkin. 2017. "Secular and Race/Ethnic Trends in Glycemic Outcomes by BMI in US Adults: The Role of Waist Circumference." *Diabetes/Metabolism Research and Reviews* 33:e2889.

Barker, D. J. 1990. "The Fetal and Infant Origins of Adult Disease." *BMJ* 301 (6761): 1111.

Begg, D., S. Fischer, and R. Dornbusch. 2000. *Economics*. London: McGraw-Hill Companies.

Bell, C. A., L. S. Adair, and B. M. Popkin. 2002. "Ethnic Differences in the Association between Body Mass Index and Hypertension." *American Journal of Epidemiology* 155 (4): 346–53.

Bray, G., K. Kim, J. Wilding, and World Obesity Federation. 2017. "Obesity: A Chronic Relapsing Progressive Disease Process. A Position Statement of the World Obesity Federation." *Obesity Reviews* 18 (7): 715–23.

Cawley, J., and C. Meyerhoefer. 2012. "The Medical Care Costs of Obesity: An Instrumental Variables Approach." *Journal of Health Economics* 31 (1): 219–30.

Chaudri, R., and C. P. Timmer. 1986. "The Impact of Changing Affluence on Diet and Demand Patterns for Agricultural Commodities." Staff Working Paper 785, World Bank, Washington, DC.

Cutler, D. M., E. L. Glaeser, and J. M. Shapiro. 2003. "Why Have Americans Become More Obese?" *Journal of Economic Perspectives* 17 (3): 93–118.

Deaton, A., and J. Muellbauer. 1980. "An Almost Ideal Demand System." *American Economic Review* 70 (3): 312.

Dee, A., A. Callinan, E. Doherty, C. O'Neill, T. McVeigh, M. R. Sweeney, A. Staines, K. Kearns, S. Fitzgerald, L. Sharp, F. Kee, J. Hughes, K. Balanda, and I. J. Perry. 2015. "Overweight and Obesity on the Island of Ireland: An Estimation of Costs." *BMJ Open* 5:e006189.

Delgado, C. L. 2003. "Rising Consumption of Meat and Milk in Developing Countries Has Created a New Food Revolution." *Journal of Nutrition* 133 (11 Suppl 2): 3907S–3910S.

Delgado, C., M. Rosegrant, H. Steinfield, S. Ehui, and C. Courbois. 1999. "Livestock to 2020: The Next Food Revolution." Food, Agriculture, and the Environment Discussion Paper 28, International Food Policy Research Institute, Washington, DC.

Dobbs, R., C. Sawers, F. Thompson, J. Manyika, J. Woetzel, P. Child, S. McKenna, and A. Spatharou. 2014. "Overcoming Obesity: An Initial Economic Analysis." McKinsey Global Institute Discussion Paper. https://www.mckinsey.com /~/media/McKinsey/Business%20Functions/Economic%20Studies%20TEMP /Our%20Insights/How%20the%20world%20could%20better%20fight%20 obesity/MGI_Overcoming_obesity_Full_report.ashx.

Drewnowski, A., and S. E. Specter. 2004. "Poverty and Obesity: The Role of Energy Density and Energy Cost." *American Journal of Clinical Nutrition* 79: 6–16.

Duffey, K. J., R. A. Pereira, and B. M. Popkin. 2013. "Prevalence and Energy Intake from Snacking in Brazil: Analysis of the First Nationwide Individual Survey." *European Journal of Clinical Nutrition* 67 (8): 868–74.

Duffey, K. J., J. A. Rivera, and B. M. Popkin. 2014. "Snacking Is Prevalent in Mexico." *Journal of Nutrition* 144 (11): 1843–49.

Dunford, E. K., and B. M. Popkin. 2017. "37 Year Snacking Trends for US Children 1977-2014." *Pediatric Obesity* 13 (4): 247–55.

EAT *Lancet* Commission. 2019. Willett, W., J. Rockström, B. Loken, M. Springmann, T. Lang, S. Vermeulen, T. Garnett, D. Tilman, F. DeClerck, A. Wood, M. Jonell, M. Clark, L. J. Gordon, J. Fanzo, C. Hawkes, R. Zurayk, J. A. Rivera, W. De Vries, L. Majele Sibanda, A. Afshin, A. Chaudhary, M. Herrero, R. Agustina, F. Branca, A. Lartey, S. Fan, B. Crona, E. Fox, V. Bignet, M. Troell, T. Lindahl, S. Singh, S. E. Cornell, K. Srinath Reddy, S. Narain, S. Nishtar, and C. J. L. Murray. "Food in the Anthropocene: The EAT–Lancet Commission on Healthy

Diets from Sustainable Food Systems." *The Lancet* 393 (10170): 447–92. https://www.thelancet.com/commissions/EAT.

Emery, C., J. Dinet, A. Lafuma, C. Sermet, B. Khoshnood, and F. Fagnani. 2007. "Cost of Obesity in France." *La Presse Médicale* 36 (6 Pt 1): 832–40.

Epstein, L. H., N. Jankowiak, C. Nederkoom, H. A. Raynor, S. A. French, and E. Finkelstein. 2012. "Experimental Research on the Relation between Food Price Changes and Food-Purchasing Patterns: A Targeted Review." *American Journal of Clinical Nutrition* 95 (4):789–809.

Ercin, A. E., M. M. Aldaya, and A. Y. Hoekstra. 2011. "Corporate Water Footprint Accounting and Impact Assessment: The Case of the Water Footprint of a Sugar-Containing Carbonated Beverage." *Water Resources Management* 25 (2): 721–41.

Erlanson-Albertsson, C., and R. Zetterstrom. 2005. "The Global Obesity Epidemic: Snacking and Obesity May Start with Free Meals during Infant Feeding." *Acta Paediatrica* 94 (11): 1523–31.

FAO (Food and Agriculture Organization of the United Nations). 2007. *Livestock's Long Shadow: Environmental Issues and Options.* Rome: FAO.

Finkelstein, E. A., D. S. Brown, D. R. Brown, and D. M. Buchner. 2008. "A Randomized Study of Financial Incentives to Increase Physical Activity among Sedentary Older Adults." *Preventive Medicine* 47 (2): 182–87.

Finkelstein, E. A., I. C. Fiebelkorn, and G. Wang. 2003. "National Medical Spending Attributable to Overweight and Obesity: How Much, and Who's Paying?" *Health Affairs (Millwood)* 22 (3): 219–26.

Finkelstein, E. A., and K. L. Strombotne. 2010. "The Economics of Obesity." *American Journal of Clinical Nutrition* 91 (5): 1520S–1524S.

Finkelstein, E. A., J. G. Trogdon, J. W. Cohen, and W. Dietz. 2009. "Annual Medical Spending Attributable to Obesity: Payer- and Service-Specific Estimates." *Health Affairs* 28 (5): 822–31.

GBD 2015 Obesity Collaborators. 2017. "Health Effects of Overweight and Obesity in 195 Countries over 25 Years." *New England Journal of Medicine* 377 (1): 13–27.

Godfray, H. C. J., P. Aveyard, T. Garnett, J. W. Hall, T. J. Key, J. Lorimer, R. T. Pierrehumbert, P. Scarborough, M. Springmann, and S. A. Jebb. 2018. "Meat Consumption, Health, and the Environment." *Science* 361 (6399).

Goettler, A., A. Grosse, and D. Sonntag. 2017. "Productivity Loss Due to Overweight and Obesity: A Systematic Review of Indirect Costs." *BMJ Open* 2017; 7:e014632.

Gordon-Larsen, P., S. M. Attard, A. G. Howard, B. M. Popkin, B. Zhang, S. Du, and D. K. Guilkey. 2017. "Accounting for Selectivity Bias and Correlation across the Sequence from Elevated Blood Pressure to Hypertension Diagnosis and Treatment." *American Journal of Hypertension* 31 (1): 63–71.

Guh, D. P., W. Zhang, N. Bansback, Z. Amarsi, C. L. Birmingham, and A. H. Anis. 2009. "The Incidence of Co-Morbidities Related to Obesity and Overweight: A Systematic Review and Meta-Analysis." *BMC Public Health* 9 (1): 88.

Herrin, A. N. 1979. "Rural Electrification and Fertility Change in the Southern Philippines." *Population and Development Review* 5: 61–86.

Hoekstra, A. Y. 2013. *The Water Footprint of Modern Consumer Society.* Oxon, UK, and New York: Routledge.

Hoekstra, A. Y. and A. K. Chapagain. 2007. "Water Footprints of Nations: Water Use by People as a Function of Their Consumption Pattern." *Water Resources Management* 21: 35–48.

House of Commons Health Select Committee. 2004. *Obesity: Third Report of Session 2003/2004.* The Stationery Office: London. http://www.sbu.se/upload/Publikationer /Content0/1/obesity_2002/obsesityslut.pdf.

Huffman, S. L., E. G. Piwoz, S. A. Vosti, and K. G. Dewey. 2014. "Babies, Soft Drinks and Snacks: A Concern in Low- and Middle-Income Countries?" *Maternal and Child Nutrition* 10 (4): 562–74.

Kang, J. H., B. G. Jeong, Y. G. Cho, H. R. Song, and K. A. Kim. 2011. "Socioeconomic Costs of Overweight and Obesity in Korean Adults." *Journal of Korean Medical Science* 26 (12): 1533–40.

Katzmarzyk, P. T., and I. Janssen. 2004. "The Economic Costs Associated with Physical Inactivity and Obesity in Canada: An Update." *Canadian Journal of Applied Physiology* 29: 90–115.

Konnopka, A., M. Bödemann, and H. H. König. 2011. "Health Burden and Costs of Obesity and Overweight in Germany." *European Journal of Health Economics* 12 (4): 345–52.

Kosen, S. 2018. "The Economic Burden of Overweight and Obesity Reaches 3% of GDP in Indonesia." *Asia Pathways* blog post, February 2. https://www .asiapathways-adbi.org/2018/02/the-economic-burden-of-overweight-and -obesity-in-indonesia/.

Kuzawa, C., P. C. Hallal, L. Adair, S. K. Bhargava, C. H. Fall, N. Lee, S. A. Norris, C. Osmond, P. M. Ramirez-Zea, H. S. Sachdev, A. D. Stein, and C. G. Victora, and COHORTS Group. 2011. "Birth Weight, Postnatal Weight Gain and Adult Body Composition in Five Low and Middle Income Countries." *American Journal of Human Biology* 24 (1): 5–13.

Kyle, T. K., E. J. Dhurandhar, and D. B. Allison. 2016. "Regarding Obesity as a Disease: Evolving Policies and Their Implications." *Endocrinology and Metabolism Clinics of North America* 45 (3): 511–20.

Law, C. M., D. J. Barker, C. Osmond, C. H. Fall, and S. J. Simmonds. 1992. "Early Growth and Abdominal Fatness in Adult Life." *Journal of Epidemiology and Community Health* 46 (3): 184–86.

LCO (*Lancet* Commission on Obesity). 2019. Swinburn, B. A., V. I. Kraak, S. Allender, V. J Atkins, P. I. Baker, J. R. Bogard, H. Brinsden, A. Calvillo, O. De Schutter, R. Devarajan, M. Ezzati, S. Friel, S. Goenka, R. A. Hammond, G. Hastings, C. Hawkes, M. Herrero, P. S. Hovmand, M. Howden, L. M. Jaacks, A. B. Kapetanaki, M. Kasman, H. V. Kuhnlein, S. K. Kumanyika, B. Larijani, T. Lobstein, M. W. Long, V. K. R. Matsudo, S. D. H. Mills, G. Morgan, A. Morshed, P. M. Nece, A. Pan, D. W. Patterson, G. Sacks, M. Shekar, G. L. Simmons, W. Smit, A. Tootee, S. Vandevijvere, W. E. Waterlander, L. Wolfenden, and W. H. Dietz. 2019. "The Global Syndemic of Obesity, Undernutrition, and Climate Change: The Lancet Commission Report." *The Lancet* 393 (10173): 791–846. https://www.thelancet.com/commissions /global-syndemic.

Lehnert, T., P. Streltchenia, A. Konnopka, S. G. Riedel-Heller, and H.-H. Konig. 2015. "Health Burden and Costs of Obesity and Overweight in Germany: An Update." *European Journal of Health Economics* 16: 957–67.

Lobstein, T., H. Brinsden, T. Gill, S. Kumanyika, and B. Swinburn. 2017. "Comment: Obesity as a Disease – Some Implications for the World Obesity Federation's Advocacy and Public Health Activities." *Obesity Reviews* 18 (7): 724–26.

Martin-Rodriguez, E., F. Guillen-Grima, A. Martí, and A. Brugos-Larumbe. 2015. "Comorbidity Associated with Obesity in a Large Population: The APNA Study." *Obesity Research and Clinical Practice* 9 (5): 435–47.

Monteiro, C. A., J. C. Moubarac, G. Cannon, S. W. Ng, and B. Popkin. 2013. "Ultra-Processed Products Are Becoming Dominant in the Global Food System." *Obesity Reviews* 14 (S2): 21–28.

Ng, S. W., E. C. Norton, D. K. Guilkey, and B. M. Popkin. 2012. "Estimation of a Dynamic Model of Weight." *Empirical Economics* 42 (2): 413–43.

Ng, S. W., E. C. Norton, and B. M. Popkin. 2009. "Why Have Physical Activity Levels Declined among Chinese Adults? Findings from the 1991–2006 China Health and Nutrition Surveys." *Social Science and Medicine* 68 (7): 1305–14.

Ng, S. W., and B. M. Popkin. 2012. "Time Use and Physical Activity: A Shift Away from Movement across the Globe." *Obesity Reviews* 13 (8): 659–80.

Popkin, B. M. 2008. *The World Is Fat: The Fads, Trends, Policies, and Products That Are Fattening the Human Race*. New York: Avery-Penguin Group.

———. 2011. "Agricultural Policies, Food and Public Health." *EMBO Reports* 12 (1): 11–18.

———. 2014. "Nutrition, Agriculture and the Global Food System in Low and Middle Income Countries." *Food Policy* 47: 91–96.

Popkin, B. M., S. Kim, E. R. Rusev, S. Du, and C. Zizza. 2006. "Measuring the Full Economic Costs of Diet, Physical Activity and Obesity-Related Chronic Diseases." *Obesity Reviews* 7: 271–93.

Popkin, B. M., and T. Reardon. 2018. "Obesity and the Food System Transformation in Latin America." *Obesity Reviews* 19 (8): 1028–64.

Pries, A. M., A. M. Rehman, S. Filteau, N. Sharma, A. Upadhyay, and E. L. Ferguson. 2019. "Unhealthy Snack Food and Beverage Consumption Is Associated with Lower Dietary Adequacy and Length-for-Age z-Scores among 12–23-Month-Olds in Kathmandu Valley, Nepal." *Journal of Nutrition* 149 (10): 1843–51.

Qin, X., and J. Pan. 2016. "The Medical Cost Attributable to Obesity and Overweight in China: Estimation Based on Longitudinal Surveys." *Health Economics* 25 (10): 1291–311.

Reardon, T., C. P. Timmer, C. B. Barrett, and J. A. Berdegue. 2003. "The Rise of Supermarkets in Africa, Asia, and Latin America." *American Journal of Agricultural Economics* 85: 1140–46.

Roester, N. 2017. "Global Savory Snack Market Ripe for Growth." *Food Business News,* April 7. https://www.foodbusinessnews.net/articles/9167-global-savory-snack-market-ripe-for-growth.

Rtveladze, K., T. Marsh, L. Webber, F. Kilpi, D. Levy, W. Conde, K. McPherson, and M. Brown. 2013. "Health and Economic Burden of Obesity in Brazil." *PLOS ONE* 8 (7): e68785.

Seabrook, J. 2011. "Snacks for a Fat Planet: PepsiCo Takes Stock of the Obesity Epidemic." *The New Yorker.* May 16.

Song, H. J., J. Hwang, S. Pi, S. Ahn, Y. Heo, S. Park, and J.-W. Kwon. 2018. "The Impact of Obesity and Overweight on Medical Expenditures and Disease Incidence in Korea from 2002 to 2013." *PLOS ONE* 13 (5): e0197057.

Springmann, M., M. Clark, D. Mason-D'Croz, K. Wiebe, B. L. Bodirsky, L. Lassaletta, W. de Vries, S. J. Vermeulen, M. Herrero, K. M. Carlson, M. Jonell, M. Troell, F. DeClerck, L. J. Gordon, R. Zurayk, P. Scarborough, M. Rayner, B. Loken,

J. Fanzo, H. C. J. Godfray, D. Tilman, J. Rockström, and W. Willett. 2018. "Options for Keeping the Food System within Environmental Limits." *Nature* 562 (7728): 519–25.

Stein, A. D., M. Wang, R. Martorell, S. A. Norris, L. S. Adair, I. Bas, H. S. Sachdev, S. K. Bhargava, C. H. Fall, D. P. Gigante, and C. G. Victora. 2010. "Growth Patterns in Early Childhood and Final Attained Stature: Data from Five Birth Cohorts from Low- and Middle-Income Countries." *American Journal of Human Biology* 22 (3): 353–59.

Swedish Council on Technology Assessment in Health Care. 2002. "Obesity – Problems and Interventions: A Systematic Review." http://www.sbu.se/upload /Publikationer/Content0/1/obesity_2002/obsesityslut.pdf.

Timmer, C. P., and H. Alderman. 1979. "Estimating Consumption Parameters for Food Policy Analysis." *American Journal of Agricultural Economics* 61 (5): 982–87.

Tremmel, M., U. G. Gerdthan, P. M. Nilsson, and S. Saha. 2017. "Economic Burden of Obesity: A Systematic Literature Review." *International Journal of Environmental Research and Public Health* 14 (4): 435.

Tschirley, D., T. Reardon, M. Dolislager, and J. Snyder. 2015. "The Rise of a Middle Class in East and Southern Africa: Implications for Food System Transformation." *Journal of International Development* 27 (5): 628–46.

Vazquez-Sanchez, R., and J., Lam. 2002. "Obesity Costs Reach 7% of Total Health Care Expenses." *Revista Española de Salud Pública* 1 (3): 40–42.

Victora, C. G., L. Adair, C. Fall, P. C. Hallal, R. Martorell, L. Richter, and H. S. Sachdev. 2008. "Maternal and Child Undernutrition: Consequences for Adult Health and Human Capital." *The Lancet* 371 (9609): 340–57.

Wang, Z., F. Zhai, B. Zhang, and B. M. Popkin. 2012. "Trends in Chinese Snacking Behaviors and Patterns and the Social-Demographic Role between 1991 and 2009." *Asia Pacific Journal of Clinical Nutrition* 21 (2): 253–62.

Waters, H., and M. Graf. 2018. *America's Obesity Crisis: The Health and Economic Costs of Excess Weight.* Santa Monica, CA: Milken Institute. https://assets1c .milkeninstitute.org/assets/Publication/ResearchReport/PDF/Mi-Americas -Obesity-Crisis-WEB.pdf.

WCRF and AICR (World Cancer Research Fund and American Institute for Cancer Research). 2018. *Diet, Nutrition, Physical Activity and Cancer: A Global Perspective (A Summary of the Third Expert Report).* Continuous Update Project Expert Report 2018. London: WCRF. https://www.wcrf.org/sites/default/files/Summary -third-expert-report.pdf.

Wells, J. C. K., R. Wibaek, and M. Poullas. 2018. "The Dual Burden of Malnutrition Increases the Risk of Cesarean Delivery: Evidence From India." *Frontiers in Public Health* 6: 292.

WHO (World Health Organization) Expert Consultation. 2004. "Appropriate Body-Mass Index for Asian Populations and Its Implications for Policy and Intervention Strategies." *The Lancet* 363 (9403): 157–63.

WHO Western Pacific Region. 2000. *The Asian-Pacific Perspective: Redefining Obesity and Its Treatment.* Caulfield, Victoria: International Diabetes Institute.

Zhai, F. Y., S. F. Du, Z. H. Wang, J. G. Zhang, W. W. Du, and B. M. Popkin. 2014. "Dynamics of the Chinese Diet and the Role of Urbanicity, 1991–2011." *Obesity Reviews* 15: 16–26.

4

Factors Affecting Overweight/Obesity Prevalence

Barry Popkin, Julia Dayton Eberwein, and Kyoko Shibata Okamura

Key Messages

- Three sets of factors can affect overweight/obesity: (1) early life undernutrition and reduced linear growth, (2) reduced energy expenditure through changes in technology and lifestyles in all phases of life, and (3) a set of factors linked to changing food systems and the resultant shifts in food consumption and eating behaviors.
- Urbanization has been a major global factor affecting overweight/obesity because of the confluence of changes wrought by urban living that affect both diet and activity patterns.
- Globalization—particularly the free trade of services such as modern marketing trade in food products as well as methods of production and retailing—has been another global factor in speeding the growth of overweight/obesity.
- Country wealth, as seen in increased national income as well as increased household income, has been linked to higher rates of overweight/obesity. Similarly, greater female labor force participation has played a critical role in the shift toward greater consumption of convenient, time-saving, ultra-processed food.

- Modern food retail and food service systems are growing rapidly in low- and middle-income countries. Around the world, more television ads are placed for unhealthy foods and drinks than for healthy ones, especially during children's peak viewing times. Further, marketers now have much more tools, such as mobile, viral, and social media, to target young audiences. With these modern systems and aggressive marketing come rapid increases in consumption of ultra-processed foods, shown to be highly obesogenic. Increased consumption of ultra-processed foods may be one of the major global factors affecting overweight/obesity today.
- At the individual level, lifestyle changes and modern energy-saving technologies—in the home, in the workplace, in the use of personal cars and motorcycles as a mode of transportation, and through modern urban design—have significantly reduced physical activity. Reduced physical activity and increased sedentary behavior likely represent the most important causes of the rapid overweight/obesity increases that occurred between 1990 and 2010 in most low- and middle-income countries.

Figure 4.1 Factors Affecting Overweight/Obesity: A Conceptual Framework

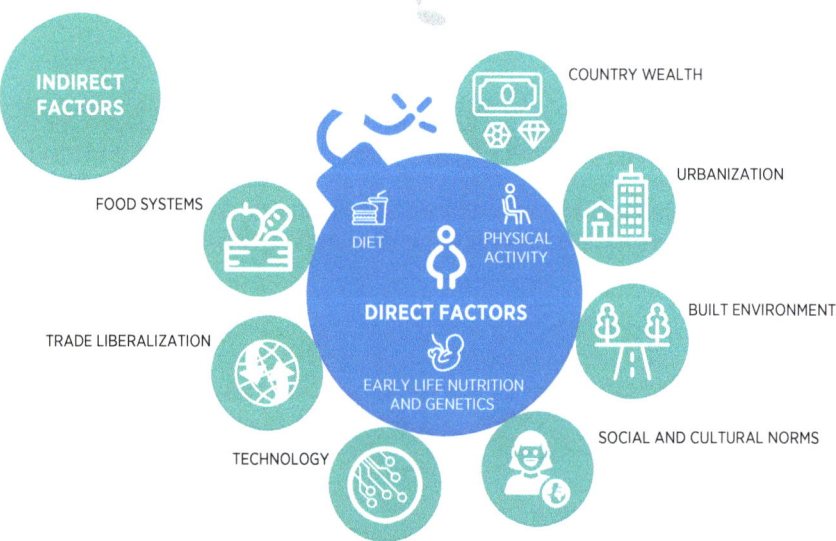

The key factors affecting overweight/obesity as laid out in the conceptual framework (figure 4.1) are discussed in depth in this chapter.

Global Factors Associated with Increased Overweight/Obesity

An array of studies and reviews has repeatedly found that overweight and obesity are linked closely to urbanization and the globalization of access to goods and services and modern technologies. One of the first major documents concerned with the global situation was a World Health Organization (WHO) report addressing the obesity epidemic in 2000, followed by the second report in 2002 (WHO 2000; Joint WHO/FAO Expert Consultation 2002). These represent the beginning of global recognition of this rapid increase in overweight/obesity in all countries. Most of the increase in overweight/obesity in low- and middle-income countries' occurred in urban areas, so this was a major focus of research and policy discussions (Popkin 1999). The literature on urbanization is vast, with documentation of major shifts in activity patterns, access to modern food supply, and new lifestyles (Jones-Smith and Popkin 2010; Monda et al. 2007; Popkin 1999; Popkin and Reardon 2018). Globalization was a second major factor, and included open access to modern technologies affecting both activity and dietary patterns (Clark et al. 2012; Hawkes and Thow 2008; Thow and Hawkes 2009).

Urbanization. The urbanization literature shows that a confluence of components that define urbanization—modern transportation, more service sector jobs, access to modern technology in factories, modern communications, water and public infrastructure, housing, higher wages, increased food services, and modern food retailing—has created an environment conducive to overweight/obesity. Extensive research has shown that urban areas have had and continue to have higher overweight/obesity levels, among both adults and children (Neuman et al. 2013). This is predicted to shift in the future according to the recent report by the NCD Risk Factor Collaboration showing that faster rates of increase in adult BMI have been seen in rural areas than in urban ones in all regions except in Sub-Saharan Africa (NCD-RisC 2019).

Globalization. The globalization and trade literature is much less focused (Bogin et al. 2014; Fox, Feng, and Asal 2019; Popkin 2006; Reardon, Stamoulis, and Pingali 2007; Snowdon and Thow 2013; Thow 2009; Thow and Hawkes 2009; Wilkinson 2004). Globalization is very much represented by the increased flow of goods (for example, food retailers selling ultra-processed food), services, and technology, all of which are discussed below. In some ways, the impact of urbanization showed the initial effects of globalization on overweight/obesity. The other effects of globalization are covered by many of the factors noted below, ranging from the population's access to the modern food sector to technology affecting all aspects of activity and modern food marketing as well as media penetration in every low- and middle-income country.

Country wealth. Many studies using a variety of data have shown how country wealth is related to higher body mass index and overweight/obesity (Masood and Reidpath 2017). At the same time, an array of studies show that, as country wealth increases, there are more rural poor than urban poor and the likelihood that overweight prevalence is greater among the poor than the rich increases (Jaacks, Slining, and Popkin 2015; Jones-Smith et al. 2011, 2012a, 2012b; NCD-RisC 2019; Popkin and Slining 2013).

Modern food retail sector. A substantial factor affecting overweight/obesity has been a major shift in the type of food and beverages sold by retailers including ready-to-eat, ready-to-heat, processed and packaged food (Poti et al. 2015). The past 60 years have seen a revolution in food science and in the manufacturing of highly processed foods, increasingly labeled *ultra-processed foods* in the literature. The proportion of calories obtained from these foods—which are full of additives that enhance flavors and scents and are high in added saturated fat, added sugar, and added salt—has shown explosive growth first in the 1970 to 2000 period in high-income countries, then in Latin America in the 1990s with modern retailing, and now across all remaining low- and middle-income countries (Monteiro et al. 2013; Monteiro et al. 2017; Popkin and Reardon 2018). Over the past 25 years, the availability and sales of these same ultra-processed foods have exploded across all low- and middle-income countries and all regions of the world; a growing set of studies is measuring this shift. More profoundly, there is now a solid and growing link between the shift from real foods to these ultra-processed foods and their effects on overweight/obesity as well as on many diet-related NCDs. A recent randomized controlled trial by a team of U.S. National Institutes of Health researchers, with a cross-over design where each person was his/her own control, showed that normal-weight adults fed a real food diet and then a diet composed of ultra-processed foods lost 0.9 kilograms in two weeks when fed the real food but gained 2.1 kilograms when fed the ultra-processed diet. Each group started with one diet regimen and then shifted to the other (Hall 2019). This work was further amplified by several papers in the *British Medical Journal* that looked at two large European cohorts and showed a strong positive relation between ultra-processed foods and cardiovascular disease and all-cause mortality (Lawrence and Baker 2019; Rico-Campà et al. 2019; Srour et al. 2019). There are now studies documenting the rapid growth of these ultra-processed foods in all continents among almost all low- and middle-income countries. It is the rapid growth of the sales of these foods in low- and middle-income countries that greatly threatens to increase overweight/obesity as well as undernutrition because infants are increasingly being fed these products. We are beginning to see the emergence of studies that associate these same ultra-processed foods with reduced length-for-age (Pries et al. 2019).

Lifestyle changes. A series of changes in technology and transportation infrastructure affect individual physical activity patterns and have led to massive declines in physical activity as noted below. At the same time, shifts in female labor force participation and modern food sector marketing have all combined to shift diets toward ready-to-eat or ready-to-heat convenient ultra-processed foods. The following sections provide background on these lifestyle changes and their impact. Together all these factors have profoundly affected social and cultural norms, including food norms, globally.

Technological change. The literature on the economic factors linked to overweight/obesity touches briefly on the role that technology plays in affecting its prevalence, but technology as an economic driver has been so critical a causal factor that it is important to explore it in greater depth. Most of the weight changes over the past three decades in low- and middle-income countries were driven first by reductions in physical activity. Technology has reduced occupation-related energy expenditure, has caused an increase in ready-to-eat food, has reduced cooking and food preparation time (for example, with rice cookers, kerosene stoves), and has reduced the need for physical activity in the home (for example, technology has provided piped-in water, refrigerators, washing machines) (Monda et al. 2008; Monda and Popkin 2005). For instance, the risk of overweight/obesity in China has more than doubled in relation to the decline in energy expenditure in each occupation; similarly, overall declines in market work–related physical activity have also been documented to be very significant not only in China but also in Brazil (Bell, Ge, and Popkin 2001; Ng et al. 2012).

Transportation infrastructure and design. Equally important has been a global shift in transportation-related physical activity as a result of modern technology: individuals have shifted from walking and biking toward using modes of motorized transportation. For example, the addition of personal cars and motorcycles to an economy (as in China) is associated with two times the overweight risk (Bell, Ge, and Popkin 2001). There has also been an increase in sedentary time, personified, again in China, by the child who spends much of his or her time watching television, studying, or playing computer games, and who experiences minimal physical activity

(Dearth-Wesley et al. 2017). Technology-driven changes to occupation- and transportation-based physical activity, as well as increased sedentary time, have led to a remarkable decline that represents over half of the energy expenditure in many low- and middle-income countries (Dearth-Wesley et al. 2017; Ng and Popkin 2012).

Income and female labor force participation. Two other major factors are increased income and greater female market labor force participation. The former is very much linked to the shift from higher overweight/obesity among higher socioeconomic status subpopulations to those with lower socioeconomic status (Jones-Smith et al. 2011, 2012b). These income effects are documented in earlier sections, including how economic growth has been linked to both rapid increases in access to labor-saving technologies in all domains of life and to modern, time-saving processed packaged foods. Female labor force participation has always been high in low- and middle-income countries, but it has increasingly seen improved wages and shifts to modern formal employment sectors. Rural nonfarm income earned by women and overall income earnings have greatly shifted the rise in women's opportunity costs of time, both in rural areas and in urban ones (Popkin and Reardon 2018). That means the demand for convenience foods, such as processed foods, has grown in rural areas just as it has in cities. The proximity of most rural households to urban areas means that packaged, processed foods are accessible and penetrate rural areas. This in turn has meant reduced time for food preparation and shopping and increased consumption of time-saving packaged processed food, much of which may be obesogenic ultra-processed food.

Marketing of ultra-processed food. The WHO and other major health organizations worldwide point to children's exposure to pervasive, unhealthy food marketing as a significant risk factor for childhood overweight/obesity (Cairns et al. 2013; CDC 2015; Ebbeling, Pawlak, and Ludwig 2002; Gearhardt et al. 2012; Lobstein et al. 2015; McGinnis, Gootman, and Kraak 2006; Montgomery and Chester 2009; PAHO 2011; Pries et al. 2019; Swinburn et al. 2011). Foods and drinks are promoted to children more than any other product type and in far greater proportion than to adults (Singh et al. 2008). Children are exposed every day to food marketing where they live, learn, and play—on television, at school and sports practice, in stores, at the movies, on mobile devices, and online (Federal Trade Commission 2012; Harris et al. 2009; McGinnis, Gootman, and Kraak 2006; Palmer and Carpenter 2006). In the United States, children ages 2–11 view roughly 13 ads a day for foods, beverages, and restaurants on television, and 12- to 17-year-old adolescents see 16.5 (Dembek, Harris, and Schwartz 2014). A 2019 study of television advertising in 22 countries around the world found, on average, four times more ads for unhealthy foods and drinks than for healthy ones during all television viewing times, and 35 percent more unhealthy food ads during children's peak viewing times (Kelly et al. 2019). While television has historically been the medium of choice to reach children, marketing via newer online, mobile, viral, and social media has exploded in recent years, offering marketers more tools to target young audiences (Cheyne et al. 2013; Common Sense Media 2014; McGinnis, Gootman, and Kraak 2006; Montgomery and Chester 2009). The majority of promoted food products are calorie dense and nutrient poor, with added sugar, saturated fat, and sodium well above recommended levels (for example, sugary breakfast cereals, soft drinks, candy, salty snacks, and fast foods) (American Heart Association 2016; Cairns et al. 2013; Federal Trade Commission 2012; Harris et al. 2009; Kelly et al. 2010; Matthews 2008; McGinnis, Gootman, and Kraak 2006; Palmer and Carpenter 2006; WHO 2010, 2016). Children are repeatedly exposed to marketing that portrays eating unhealthy foods in unlimited quantities as fun, cool, and exciting, and ultimately having only positive outcomes (Harris, Brownell, and Bargh 2009; Harris et al. 2009). Food, beverage, and restaurant industries spend billions of dollars every year to reach children with targeted marketing, and they spend millions lobbying against laws that might prevent them from doing so, demonstrating the value they see in the child market (Federal Trade Commission 2012; Hawkes 2004, 2007; Matthews 2008; Simon 2006; Wilson and Roberts 2012).

Factors Linked to Weight Gain and Overweight/Obesity at the Individual and Community Levels

The above analysis lays out the country-level factors that are associated with overweight/obesity across low- and middle-income countries over time. This section draws on prior cohort and longitudinal studies from low- and middle-income countries to detail the causes of overweight and obesity for individuals within populations. Evidence shows that three sets of factors can affect overweight/obesity: (1) early life undernutrition and reduced linear growth (see the discussion in chapter 2), (2) reduced energy expenditure through changes in technology and lifestyles in all phases of life, and (3) a set of factors linked to changing food systems and the resultant shifts in food consumption and eating behaviors. The literature on urbanization, access to modern technology affecting all aspects of energy expenditure, increased income, and greater female labor force participation has been reviewed above. The only area deserving of special attention is the new driver of most weight gain globally, namely the food system dynamics.

The Role of Changing Diets and Food Systems

To summarize where the globe is right now we need to understand that much of the impact of globalization and technology changes in reducing activity has taken place in most countries aside from a select few, mainly in Sub-Saharan Africa and South Asia, while the food system and its effects on diet have become a major global factor linked with increased overweight and obesity in all countries. While dietary changes—relative to declines in physical activity—may not have explained increases in overweight/obesity in the past (for example, in 1990–2010), the increased availability and consumption of ultra-processed foods and sugar-sweetened beverages, especially ready-to-eat snack foods, explain much of the recent overweight/obesity increases (2010–present) (Monteiro et al. 2011; Monteiro et al. 2013; Popkin and Hawkes 2015; Popkin and Reardon 2018). It is not only these unhealthy foods and beverages but also the large upsurge in edible oil intake in low- and middle-income countries that represents an additional element of dietary change that has uniquely impacted overweight/obesity prevalence in these contexts (Drewnowski and Popkin 1997). More recently (2000–present), the consumption of vegetable oils in low- and middle-income countries has been linked to the reduced cost of palm oil (Fitzherbert et al. 2008). At the same time, shifts away from traditional diets, which are largely composed of staple foods, have impacted over-weight/obesity prevalence in low- and middle-income countries. These dietary issues deserve consideration when identifying and designing future interventions to reduce weight gain because implementing food policies to help people change their dietary choices is much more feasible than mov-ing backward in order to reduce the use of technologies linked to labor, home, and transportation. Two recent World Bank studies laid out many of these challenges to the food system (Htenas, Tanimichi-Hoberg, and Brown 2017; Townsend et al. 2016).

Examples at the individual level of the impact of improved access to modern technology for market and home production and transportation represent critical aspects of the effects of globalization. Equally significant has been the spread of modern global and regional food retailers into most low- and middle-income countries and the ways these food retail systems have become a major part of the global transformation of food systems and subsequently diets. Reardon and others have documented across Asia, Africa, and Latin America the ways the World Trade Organization (WTO) and earlier global trade agreements allowed for free movement of food companies and retailers, resulting in the increasingly rapid transformation of global food systems (Hu et al. 2004; Popkin and Reardon 2018; Reardon et al. 2015; Reardon and Berdegué 2002; Reardon, Timmer, and Minten 2012).

Impetus for Action

Overall the literature shows that there are three sets of factors affecting overweight/obesity: early life undernutrition and reduced linear growth, reduced energy expenditure due to technological development and lifestyle changes, and shifts in food consumption and eating behaviors driven by changing food systems. Modern shifts in access to labor-saving technology and the resulting decreases in energy expenditure, along with increased food consumption and the consumption, in particular, of ultra-processed foods, have been major forces in the growth of overweight/obesity prevalence across the globe. Although changes in physical activity mostly drove the upsurge in overweight/obesity prevalence in low- and middle-income countries in the earlier periods of the endemic (1990–2010), more recently (2010–present) modern food and retail services, which are the major purveyors of ultra-processed foods and beverages, have become critical determinants of increased overweight/obesity. These shifts in energy expenditure and diet stem from greater country wealth and greater urbanization. Underlying these changes have been rapid increases in urban residency as well as a major shift in the quality of urbanization in terms of access to modern ultra-processed foods and many labor-saving technologies, global movement of goods and services, and economic growth as exemplified by real gross national product per capita, as well as large shifts in female labor force participation and female wages and thus their time costs.

As noted above, these economic and social changes were experienced by adults and adolescents much earlier than they were by younger children. In a similar way, changes in energy expenditure, along with the introduction of modern food systems, occurred first in urban areas.

Together, these results point out many critical roles that different sectors can play to help prevent the rise of overweight/obesity in future generations. Improved physical activity and reduced sedentary behavior are important for health in general as well as important to reducing overweight/obesity; however, most countries must also focus on reducing or stopping the rapid growth of consumption of ultra-processed foods.

References

American Heart Association. 2016. "Children Should Eat Less than 25 Grams of Added Sugars Daily." American Heart Association Scientific Statement News Release, August 22. https://newsroom.heart.org/news/children-should-eat-less-than-25-grams-of-added-sugars-daily.

Bell, A. C., K. Ge, and B. M. Popkin. 2001. "Weight Gain and Its Predictors in Chinese Adults." *International Journal of Obesity and Related Metabolic Disorders* 25 (7): 1079–86.

———. 2002. "The Road to Obesity or the Path to Prevention: Motorized Transportation and Obesity in China." *Obesity Research* 10 (4): 277–83.

Bogin, B., H. Azcorra, H. J. Wilson, A. Vázquez-Vázquez, M. L. Avila-Escalante, M. T. Castillo-Burguete, I. Varela-Silva, and F. Dickinson. 2014. "Globalization and Children's Diets: The Case of Maya of Mexico and Central America." *Anthropological Review* 77 (1): 11–32.

Cairns, G., K. Angus, G. Hastings, and M. Caraher. 2013. "Systematic Reviews of the Evidence on the Nature, Extent and Effects of Food Marketing to Children: A Retrospective Summary." *Appetite* 62: 209–15.

CDC (Centers for Disease Control and Prevention). 2015. "Childhood Obesity Causes & Consequences." https://www.cdc.gov/obesity/childhood/causes.html.

Cheyne, A. D., L. Dorfman, E. Bukofzer, and J. L. Harris. 2013. "Marketing Sugary Cereals to Children in the Digital Age: A Content Analysis of 17 Child-Targeted Websites." *Journal of Health Communication* 18 (5): 563–82.

Clark, S. E., C. Hawkes, S. M. Murphy, K. A. Hansen-Kuhn, and D. Wallinga. 2012. "Exporting Obesity: US Farm and Trade Policy and the Transformation of the Mexican Consumer Food Environment." *International Journal of Occupational and Environmental Health* 18 (1): 53–64.

Common Sense Media. 2014. "Advertising to Children and Teens: Current Practices." A Common Sense Media Research Brief, Common Sense Media, San Francisco. https://www.commonsensemedia.org/research/advertising-to -children-and-teens-current-practices.

Dearth-Wesley, T., A. G. Howard, H. Wang, B. Zhang, and B. M. Popkin. 2017. "Trends in Domain-Specific Physical Activity and Sedentary Behaviors among Chinese School Children, 2004–2011." *International Journal of Behavioral Nutrition and Physical Activity* 14 (1): 141.

Dembek, C., J. L. Harris, and M. B. Schwartz. 2014. "Trends in Television Food Advertising to Young People: 2013 Update." Yale Rudd Center for Food Policy and Obesity. http://www.uconnruddcenter.org/resources/upload/docs/what /reports/RuddReport_TVFoodAdvertising_6.14.pdf.

Drewnowski, A., and B. M. Popkin. 1997. "The Nutrition Transition: New Trends in the Global Diet." *Nutrition Reviews* 55 (2): 31–43.

Ebbeling, C. B., D. B. Pawlak, and D. S. Ludwig. 2002. "Childhood Obesity: Public-Health Crisis, Common Sense Cure." *The Lancet* 360 (9331): 473–82.

Federal Trade Commission. 2012. *A Review of Food Marketing to Children and Adolescents: Follow-Up Report.* Washington, DC: Federal Trade Commission. https://www.ftc .gov/sites/default/files/documents/reports/review-food-marketing-children -and-adolescents-follow-report/121221foodmarketingreport.pdf.

Fitzherbert, E. B., M. J. Struebig, A. Morel, F. Danielsen, C. A. Brühl, P. F. Donald, and B. Halan. 2008. "How Will Oil Palm Expansion Affect Biodiversity?" *Trends in Ecology and Evolution* 23 (10): 538–45.

Fox, A., W. Feng, and V. Asal. 2019. "What Is Driving Global Obesity Trends? Globalization or 'Modernization'?" *Globalization and Health* 15 (1): 32.

Gearhardt, A. N., M. A. Bragg, R. L. Pearl, N. A. Schvey, C. A. Roberto, and K. D. Brownell. 2012. "Obesity and Public Policy." *Annual Review of Clinical Psychology* 8: 405–30.

Hall, K. D. 2019. "Ultra-Processed Diets Cause Excess Calorie Intake and Weight Gain: A One-Month Inpatient Randomized Controlled Trial of Ad Libitum Food Intake." NutriXiv Preprints. Febrary 11. https://osf.io/preprints/nutrixiv /w3zh2.

Harris, J. L., K. D. Brownell, and J. A. Bargh. 2009. "The Food Marketing Defense Model: Integrating Psychological Research to Protect Youth and Inform Public Policy." *Social Issues and Policy Review* 3 (1): 211–71.

Harris, J. L., J. L. Pomeranz, T. Lobstein, and K. D. Brownell. 2009. "A Crisis in the Marketplace: How Food Marketing Contributes to Childhood Obesity and What Can Be Done." *Annual Review of Public Health* 30: 211–25.

Hawkes, C. 2004. "Marketing Food to Children." The Regulatory Framework. World Health Organization, Geneva.

———. 2007. "Regulating and Litigating in the Public Interest: Regulating Food Marketing to Young People Worldwide: Trends and Policy Drivers." *American Journal of Public Health* 97 (11): 1962–73.

Hawkes, C. and A. Thow. 2008. "Implications of the Central America-Dominican Republic-Free Trade Agreement for the Nutrition Transition in Central America." *Revista Panamericana de Salud Pública* 24 (5): 345–60.

Htenas, A. M., Y. Tanimichi-Hoberg, and L. Brown. 2017. *An Overview of Links between Obesity and Food Systems: Implications for the Agriculture GP Agenda.* Washington, DC: World Bank Group.

Hu, D., T. Reardon, S. Rozelle, P. Timmer, and H. Wang. 2004. "The Emergence of Supermarkets with Chinese Characteristics: Challenges and Opportunities for China's Agricultural Development." *Development Policy Review* 22: 557–86.

Jaacks, L. M., M. M. Slining, and B. M. Popkin. 2015. "Recent Underweight and Overweight Trends by Rural-Urban Residence among Women in Low- and Middle-Income Countries." *Journal of Nutrition* 145 (2): 352–57.

Joint WHO/FAO Expert Consultation. 2002. *Diet, Nutrition and the Prevention of Chronic Diseases: Report of a Joint WHO/FAO Expert Consultation.* Geneva: WHO.

Jones-Smith, J. C., P. Gordon-Larsen, A. Siddiqi, and B. M. Popkin. 2011. "Cross-National Comparisons of Time Trends in Overweight Inequality by Socioeconomic Status among Women Using Repeated Cross-Sectional Surveys from 37 Developing Countries, 1989–2007." *American Journal of Epidemiology* 173 (6): 667–75.

———. 2012a. "Emerging Disparities in Overweight by Educational Attainment in Chinese Adults (1989–2006)." *International Journal of Obesity* 36 (6): 866–75.

———. 2012b. "Is the Burden of Overweight Shifting to the Poor across the Globe? Time Trends among Women in 39 Low- and Middle-Income Countries (1991–2008)." *International Journal of Obesity* 36 (8): 1114–20.

Jones-Smith, J. C., and B. M. Popkin. 2010. "Understanding Community Context and Adult Health Changes in China: Development of an Urbanicity Scale." *Social Science and Medicine* 71 (8): 1436–46.

Kelly, B., J. C. Halford, E. J. Boyland, K. Chapman, I. Bautista-Castaño, C. Berg, M. Caroli, B. Cook, J. G. Coutinho, and T. Effertz. 2010. "Television Food Advertising to Children: A Global Perspective." *American Journal of Public Health* 100 (9): 1730–36.

Kelly, B., S. Vandevijvere, S. Ng, J. Adams, L. Allemandi, L. Bahena-Espina, S. Barquera, E. Boyland, P. Calleja, and I. C. Carmona-Garcés. 2019. "Global Benchmarking of Children's Exposure to Television Advertising of Unhealthy Foods and Beverages across 22 Countries." *Obesity Reviews*. https://doi .org/10.1111/obr.12840.

Lawrence, M. A., and P. I. Baker. 2019. "Ultra-Processed Food and Adverse Health Outcomes." *BMJ* 365: l2289.

Lobstein, T., R. Jackson-Leach, M. L. Moodie, K. D. Hall, S. L. Gortmaker, B. A. Swinburn, W. P. T. James, Y. Wang, and K. McPherson. 2015. "Child and Adolescent Obesity: Part of a Bigger Picture." *The Lancet* 385 (9986): 2510–20.

Masood, M., and D. D. Reidpath. 2017. "Effect of National Wealth on BMI: An Analysis of 206,266 Individuals in 70 Low-, Middle- and High-Income Countries." *PLOS ONE* 12 (6): e0178928-e0178928.

Matthews, A. E. 2008. "Children and Obesity: A Pan-European Project Examining the Role of Food Marketing." *European Journal of Public Health* 18 (1): 7–11.

McGinnis, J. M., J. A. Gootman, and V. I. Kraak. 2006. *Food Marketing to Children and Youth: Threat or Opportunity?* Washington, DC: National Academies Press.

Monda, K. L., L. S. Adair, F. Zhai, and B. M. Popkin. 2008. "Longitudinal Relationships between Occupational and Domestic Physical Activity Patterns and Body Weight in China." *European Journal of Clinical Nutrition* 62: 1318–25.

Monda, K. L., P. Gordon-Larsen, J. Stevens, and B. M. Popkin. 2007. "China's Transition: The Effect of Rapid Urbanization on Adult Occupational Physical Activity." *Social Science and Medicine* 64 (4): 858–70.

Monda, K. L., and B. M. Popkin. 2005. "Cluster Analysis Methods Help to Clarify the Activity-BMI Relationship of Chinese Youth." *Obesity Research* 13 (6): 1042–51.

Monteiro, C. A., R. B. Levy, R. M. Claro, I. R. de Castro, and G. Cannon. 2011. "Increasing Consumption of Ultra-Processed Foods and Likely Impact on Human Health: Evidence from Brazil." *Public Health Nutrition* 14 (1): 5–13.

Monteiro, C. A., J. C. Moubarac, G. Cannon, S. W. Ng, and B. Popkin. 2013. "Ultra-Processed Products Are Becoming Dominant in the Global Food System." *Obesity Reviews* 14 (S2): 21–28.

Monteiro, C. A., J.-C. Moubarac, R. B. Levy, D. S. Canella, M. L. d. C. Louzada, and G. Cannon. 2017. "Household Availability of Ultra-Processed Foods and Obesity in Nineteen European Countries." *Public Health Nutrition* 21 (1): 18–26.

Montgomery, K. C., and J. Chester. 2009. "Interactive Food and Beverage Marketing: Targeting Adolescents in the Digital Age." *Journal of Adolescent Health* 45 (3 Suppl): S18–29.

NCD-RisC (NCD Risk Factor Collaboration). 2019. "Rising Rural Body-Mass Index Is the Main Driver of the Global Obesity Epidemic in Adults." *Nature* 569 (7755): 260–64.

Neuman, M., I. Kawachi, S. Gortmaker, and S. V. Subramanian. 2013. "Urban-Rural Differences in BMI in Low- and Middle-Income Countries: The Role of Socioeconomic Status." *American Journal of Clinical Nutrition* 97 (2): 428–36.

Ng, S. W., E. C. Norton, D. K. Guilkey, and B. M. Popkin. 2012. "Estimation of a Dynamic Model of Weight." *Empirical Economics* 42 (2): 413–43.

Ng, S. W., and B. M. Popkin. 2012. "Time Use and Physical Activity: A Shift Away from Movement across the Globe." *Obesity Reviews* 13 (8): 659–80.

PAHO (Pan American Health Organization). 2011. *Recommendations from a Pan American Health Organization Expert Consultation on the Marketing of Food and Non-Alcoholic Beverages to Children in the Americas.* Washington, DC: PAHO.

Palmer, E., and C. Carpenter. 2006. "Food and Beverage Marketing to Children and Youth: Trends and Issues." *Media Psychology* 8 (2): 165–90.

Popkin, B. M. 1999. "Urbanization, Lifestyle Changes and the Nutrition Transition." *World Development* 27: 1905–16.

———. 2006. "Technology, Transport, Globalization and the Nutrition Transition." *Food Policy* 31 (6): 554–69.

Popkin, B. M., and C. Hawkes. 2015. "Sweetening of the Global Diet, Particularly Beverages: Patterns, Trends, and Policy Responses." *The Lancet Diabetes and Endocrinology* 4 (2): 174–86.

Popkin, B. M., and T. Reardon. 2018. "Obesity and the Food System Transformation in Latin America." *Obesity Reviews* 19 (8): 1028–64.

Popkin, B. M., and M. M. Slining. 2013. "New Dynamics in Global Obesity Facing Low- and Middle-Income Countries." *Obesity Reviews* 14 (Suppl 2): 11–20.

Poti, J. M., M. A. Mendez, S. W. Ng, and B. M. Popkin. 2015. "Is the Degree of Food Processing and Convenience Linked with the Nutritional Quality of Foods Purchased by US Households?" *American Journal of Clinical Nutrition* 99 (1): 162–71.

Pries, A. M., A. M. Rehman, S. Filteau, N. Sharma, A. Upadhyay, and E. L. Ferguson. 2019. "Unhealthy Snack Food and Beverage Consumption Is Associated with Lower Dietary Adequacy and Length-for-Age z-Scores among 12–23-Month-Olds in Kathmandu Valley, Nepal." *Journal of Nutrition.* https://doi.org/10.1093/jn/nxz140.

Reardon, T., and J. Berdegué. 2002. "The Rapid Rise of Supermarkets in Latin America: Challenges and Opportunities for Development." *Development Policy Review* 20 (4): 317–34.

Reardon, T., K. Stamoulis, and P. Pingali. 2007. "Rural Nonfarm Employment in Developing Countries in an Era of Globalization." *Agricultural Economics* 37 (s1): 173–83.

Reardon, T., C. Timmer, and B. Minten. 2012. "The Supermarket Revolution in Asia and Emerging Development Strategies to Include Small Farmers." *Proceedings of the National Academy of Sciences of the United States of America* 109 (31): 12332–37.

Reardon, T., D. Tschirley, B. Minten, S. Haggblade, S. Liverpool-Tasie, M. Dolislager, and C. Ijumba. 2015. "Transformation of African Agrifood Systems in the New Era of Rapid Urbanization and the Emergence of a Middle Class." In *Beyond a Middle Income Africa: Transforming African Economies for Sustained Growth with Rising Employment and Incomes,* edited by O. Badiane and T. Makombe. Chapter 4. ReSAKSS Annual Trends and Outlook Report 2014. Washington, DC: International Food Policy Research Institute (IFPRI). http://ebrary.ifpri.org/cdm/ref/collection/p15738coll2/id/130005.

Rico-Campà, A., M. A. Martínez-González, I. Alvarez-Alvarez, R. de Deus Mendonça, C. de la Fuente-Arrillaga, C. Gómez-Donoso, and M. Bes-Rastrollo. 2019. "Association between Consumption of Ultra-Processed Foods and All Cause Mortality: SUN Prospective Cohort Study." *British Medical Journal* 365: l1949.

Simon, M. 2006. "Can Food Companies Be Trusted to Self-Regulate: An Analysis of Corporate Lobbying and Deception to Undermine Children's Health." *Loyola of Los Angeles Law Review* 39: 169.

Singh, A. S., C. Mulder, J. W. Twisk, W. van Mechelen, and M. J. Chinapaw. 2008. "Tracking of Childhood Overweight into Adulthood: A Systematic Review of the Literature." *Obesity Reviews* 9 (5): 474–88.

Snowdon, W., and A. M. Thow. 2013. "Trade Policy and Obesity Prevention: Challenges and Innovation in the Pacific Islands." *Obesity Reviews* 14: 150–58.

Srour, B., L. K. Fezeu, E. Kesse-Guyot, B. Allès, C. Méjean, R. M. Andrianasolo, E. Chazelas, M. Deschasaux, S. Hercberg, and P. Galan. 2019. "Ultra-Processed Food Intake and Risk of Cardiovascular Disease: Prospective Cohort Study (NutriNet-Santé)." *British Medical Journal* 365: l1451.

Swinburn, B. A., G. Sacks, K. D. Hall, K. McPherson, D. T. Finegood, M. L. Moodie, and S. L. Gortmaker. 2011. "The Global Obesity Pandemic: Shaped by Global Drivers and Local Environments." *The Lancet* 378 (9793): 804–14.

Thow, A. M. 2009. "Trade Liberalisation and the Nutrition Transition: Mapping the Pathways for Public Health Nutritionists." *Public Health Nutrition* 12 (11): 2150–58.

Thow, A. M. and C. Hawkes. 2009. "The Implications of Trade Liberalization for Diet and Health: A Case Study from Central America." *Global Health* 5: 5.

Townsend, R., S. M. Jaffee, Y. Hoberg-Tanimichi, A. M. Htenas, M. Shekar, Z. Hyder, M. Gautam, H. A. Kray, L. Ronchi, S. Hussain, L. K. Elder, and E. Moses. 2016. *The Future of Food: Shaping the Global Food System to Deliver Improved Nutrition and Health.* Washington, DC: World Bank.

WHO (World Health Organization). 2000. *Obesity: Preventing and Managing the Global Epidemic. Report of a WHO Consultation.* Geneva: WHO.

———. 2010. *Set of Recommendations on the Marketing of Foods and Non-Alcoholic Beverages to Children.* Geneva: WHO.

———. 2016. *Consideration of the Evidence on Childhood Obesity for the Commission on Ending Childhood Obesity: Report of the Ad Hoc Working Group on Science and Evidence for Ending Childhood Obesity.* Geneva: WHO.

Wilkinson, J. 2004. "The Food Processing Industry, Globalization and Developing Countries." *Electronic Journal of Agricultural and Development Economics* 1(2): 184–201.

Wilson, D., and J. Roberts. 2012. "Special Report: How Washington Went Soft on Childhood Obesity." Reuters Special Reports, April 27, 2012. https://www.reuters.com/article/us-usa-foodlobby/special-report-how-washington-went-soft-on-childhood-obesity-idUSBRE83Q0ED20120427.

5

Addressing Overweight/ Obesity: Lessons for Future Actions

Barry Popkin, Pia Schneider, and Meera Shekar

Key Messages

- Fiscal policies linked mainly to sugar-sweetened beverage (SSB) taxes but also, in selected countries, ultra-processed foods have been seen as key areas for intervention. Major efforts are starting in a number of countries around food marketing at the media, retail, and product level (via front-of-package food labeling and profiling).
- Front-of-package labeling and related nutrition profiling models with warning labels show great promise for helping to shift consumption away from ultra-processed foods and beverages.
- There is now extensive global experience in designing taxation on SSBs, albeit taxation on other unhealthy foods such as ultra-processed foods has yet to become mainstream.
- Diet-related taxes remain a promising approach, although they will face challenges. The main challenges to the successful implementation of these taxes are a tax system's administrative capacity,

This chapter draws on lessons learned from nine case studies, conducted by the World Bank Health, Nutrition and Population teams, of country-level experiences with strategies to reduce overweight/obesity, supplemented with a review of the global literature.

substitution effects, tax evasion, and opposition from the food industry. These challenges need to be considered when designing effective tax policies.

- Countries with strong tax administrations generally design excise taxes based on nutrient content. Alternatively, taxes on product volumes may be easier to implement in countries where tax administration is not so strong. Tiered tax systems based on sugar consumption appear to be another promising approach. And experience suggests that a regional approach to taxation will reduce cross-border purchases and prevent tax evasion.

- No countries have considered tying diet-based taxes to subsidies for legumes, vegetables, fruits, and other healthful, less obesogenic foods. This might have potential, although the challenges of earmarking sin taxes for public programs bring even more challenges. One key thrust in many countries is removing SSBs from schools and promoting only healthy beverages to be sold or provided in school feeding programs.

- To date, no countries have tackled the rapidly growing food service sector. Nor is there much experience with subsidies for healthier foods or marketing regulation for unhealthy foods, except perhaps what has been learned from the marketing of infant formulas.

- Experience with physical activity improvements for obesity prevention is limited to a handful of countries, mostly in the global north; while these are promising strategies, future efforts need to build in evaluation of large-scale urban or national programs to document their impacts. No evaluations equivalent to the Mexican or Chilean rigorous evaluations of their food-related fiscal and regulatory policies yet exist in the physical activity domain.

- Concurrent important shifts in urban planning and design are being undertaken. All forms of design that increase physical activity—from building design that makes stairs an attractive option to active transport and urban design to incentivize and enable biking and walking—are important. Aside from climate co-benefits, there is a need to continue to build the case for this sector's impact on overall activity.

- The most neglected area is food systems, including sectoral work related to farms, agribusinesses, food retailers, and food service chains as well as street vendors. While there has been much discussion on this in the recent literature, few actionable agendas have been identified. The evidence for programmatic and policy impact remains unclear.

Typology of Actions to Prevent Overweight/Obesity

The evidence base for preventing overweight/obesity is still emerging; table 5.1 summarizes promising interventions/policies that have the potential to prevent overweight/obesity. These include a range of (1) fiscal policies such as taxation and subsidies; (2) regulatory policies on marketing and advertising; (3) food systems approaches including through food service; (4) education sector policies such as school cafeterias and physical activity in schools; (5) transport and urban design interventions such as mass transit and city and building design; and (6) early childhood nutrition programs that focus on improving breastfeeding rates and reducing stunting among children. Unlike many other public health interventions, very few of these policies or interventions have been rigorously evaluated (except for early childhood nutrition programs), and they have not been and cannot be tested through randomized controlled trials, and few have undergone systematic reviews because their effectiveness has not yet been demonstrated or carefully documented. Nonetheless, initial assessments, a limited number of systematic reviews, and lessons from several countries suggest that the following policies/interventions are promising, not just for their potential impacts on preventing overweight/obesity, but also for potential climate co-benefits. In addition, a series of interventions have been shown to impact undernutrition, such as breastfeeding promotion, that are also triple-duty actions in terms of their impact on undernutrition, overweight, and climate change.

Table 5.1 summarizes the suitability of various intervention types (see also table 5.4) in different country contexts.

Approaches to Reducing Overweight/Obesity

It is clear that the reasons for the rapid increases in overweight/obesity across low- and middle-income countries include a combination of major shifts toward reduced physical activity and increased sedentariness as well as shifts in food consumption patterns. Reducing excessive weight gain and ultimately reducing future overweight/obesity will require a multisectoral approach. Achieving these goals are critical for achieving the United Nations' Sustainable Development Goals (SDGs).

To date, much of the focus in countries with active overweight/obesity prevention programs has been exclusively on the food sector, in particular on three major spheres of activity: (1) fiscal policies mainly linked to taxation of SSBs, ultra-processed foods, and selected other unhealthy foods and beverages; (2) marketing work focused on two areas: front-of-package food labeling systems and marketing controls both for media that market directly

Table 5.1   Typology of Interventions

Intervention type	Suitable for			Notes/comments
	Low-income countries	Middle-income countries	High-income countries	
Fiscal policies	X	X	X	These policies show the most evidence of impact to date.
Regulatory policies	X	X	X	These policies show growing evidence of impact potential.
Agriculture/food systems	X	X	X	Limited or no impact evaluations on agriculture and food systems.
Education sector policies				Marketing controls are needed first before education programs can be effective.
Transport/urban design		X	X	Limited or no impact evaluations on transport shifts and their impact on physical activity.
Early childhood nutrition programs	X			These programs have the strongest evaluation base to date but are focused more on the impact on undernutrition—not overweight/obesity.

and solely to children and, more recently, for broader marketing approaches such as character branding and coverage that is wider than just child-oriented media; and (3) programs focused both on school feeding and the marketing and selling of ultra-processed foods in schools and areas around schools.

Concurrent important shifts in urban planning and design are occurring. All forms of design that increase physical activity—from building design that makes stairs an attractive option to urban design of walkable city areas; from approaches to incentivize and enable biking and walking to instigating weekend days when driving is banned in major urban areas; and from designing public transport and mass transit systems that provide an alternative to driving to plans that enhance walking and cycling to bus or subway systems—are important, albeit the impact of these strategies has not been studied.

This section reviews the lessons learned from countries that have experimented with these approaches.

First the focus is on fiscal policies: the area that has seen the most attention globally. Fiscal policies are highlighted as being among the most promising tools for governments to create incentives to encourage healthy lifestyles, promote the consumption of healthy products, and provide disincentives for the consumption of unhealthy products.

Fiscal policies include taxes to increase the price of taxed products and subsidies to decrease the price of healthier food for consumers (see table 5.2 for an overview of taxation options). The expectation is that consumers will

Table 5.2 Diet-Related Taxes in Five Case Study Areas

	Country (effective date)				
Tax type	Mexico (2014) Excise and ad valorem	Chile (2014) Ad valorem	Kerala, India (2016–17) Ad valorem	Thailand (2017) Excise and ad valorem	South Africa (2018) Excise
Tax rates on products	Mexican peso 1 per liter on any non-alcoholic drink with added sugar (rate inflated only after 10% inflation mark hit) 8% of price of energy-dense foods with >275 calories per 100 grams[a]	Raised from 13% to 18% for SSBs with >15 grams of sugar per 240 ml	Fat tax of 14.5% on unhealthy food sold in restaurants with brand name or trademark registered	Baht 0.1–1.0 per liter beverage with >6 grams of sugar per 100 ml 14% of retail price on SSB After 6 years, rate increases to 5 baht per liter for drinks with >10 grams of sugar per 100 ml beginning in 2023	Rand 2.1 cents per gram for SSB with >4 grams of sugar per 100 ml (legislation to increase the tax is currently under consideration)
Price pass-through	≈10%	≈3%	Unclear	Unclear	≈10% preliminary 6 months' analysis

Sources: Vilar-Compte 2018 (Mexico); Azar 2018 (Chile); Nair and Suresh (Kerala, India, forthcoming); for Thailand and South Africa, case study reports are being prepared by the World Bank.

Note: ml = milliliters; SSB = Sugar-sweetened beverages.
a. Energy-dense foods include snacks, confectionary products, chocolate, puddings, flans, ice cream, candies, and peanut butter.

react to price changes set by taxes and subsidies. Both aim to influence consumer behaviors at the point of purchase by encouraging consumers to purchase lower-priced foods and reduce consumption of higher-priced products. It has been estimated that a 10 percent price increase on sugary drinks through a tax would reduce consumption by about 10 percent and lead to a reduction of 20 kilocalories per day (Härkänen et al. 2014). To date, over 40 countries have added diet-related taxes on SSBs and several have also taxed unhealthy foods, with a large number of other countries considering similar proposals. The maps of countries with such taxes to date provide some sense of the range and variety of taxes (see maps 5.1–5.4). Few of these taxation approaches have been rigorously evaluated for their impact on prices, food purchases, or dietary intake. Only a select number of these taxes in low- and middle-income countries and high-income countries are being carefully evaluated.

Similarly, a government subsidy or a tax exemption policy decreases the price for consumers and can lead to increased consumption and consequently increased production to meet higher consumer demand. Subsidized food products often include rice and wheat or foods high in protein, such as pulses. Governments also exempt specific products from value added taxes (VAT) that are levied on goods and services. Not all goods are taxed: medicines, milk, bread, and other basic staples are among the goods that tend to

Map 5.1 Sugar-Sweetened Beverage Taxes around the World

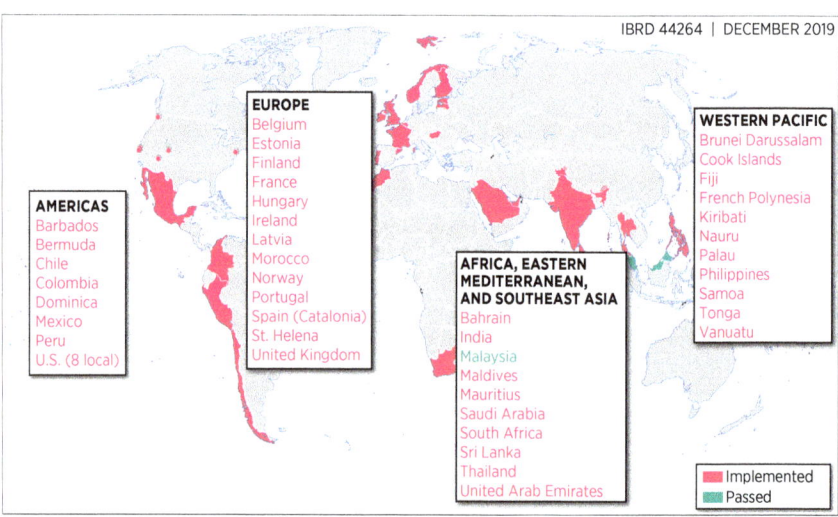

Source: Global Food Research Program, University of North Carolina, http://globalfood-researchprogram.web.unc.edu/multi-country-initiative/resources/.

Note: The map was created based on the dataset available as of March 2019.

Map 5.2 Sugar-Sweetened Beverage Taxes: The Americas

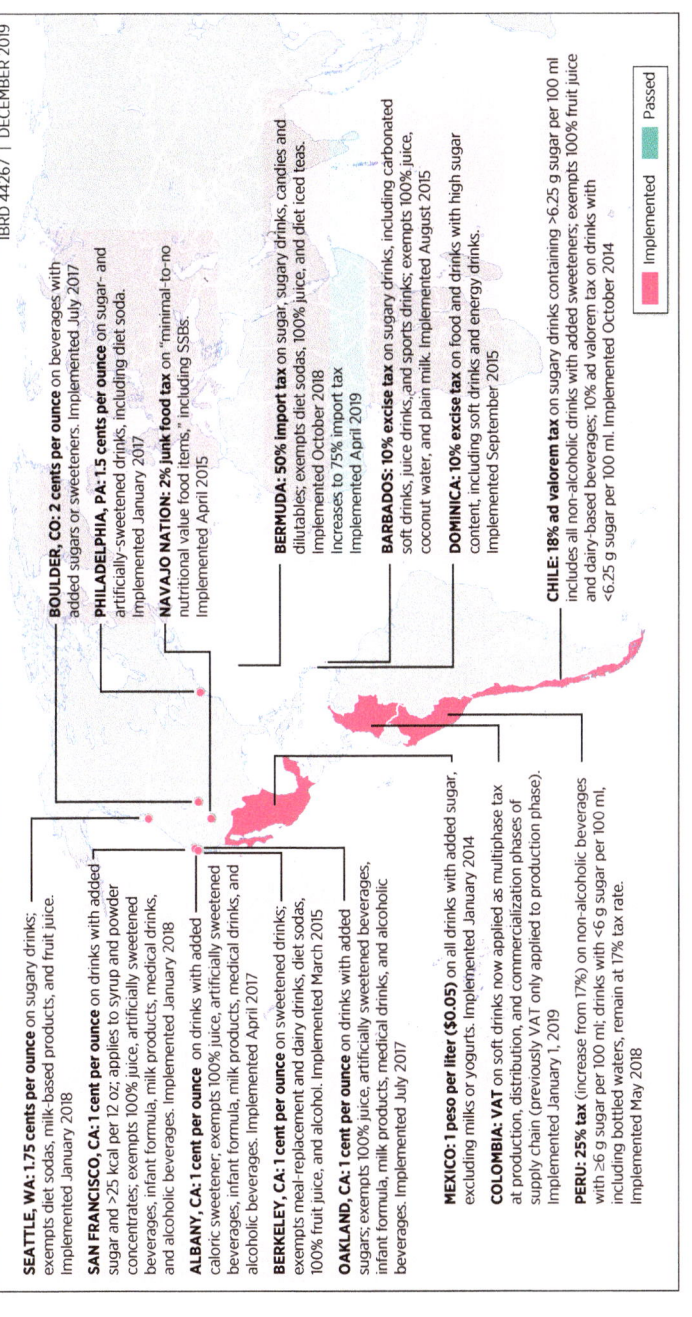

IBRD 44267 | DECEMBER 2019

SEATTLE, WA: 1.75 cents per ounce on sugary drinks; exempts diet sodas, milk-based products, and fruit juice. Implemented January 2018

SAN FRANCISCO, CA: 1 cent per ounce on drinks with added sugar and >25 kcal per 12 oz; applies to syrup and powder concentrates; exempts 100% juice, artificially sweetened beverages, infant formula, milk products, medical drinks, and alcoholic beverages. Implemented January 2018

ALBANY, CA: 1 cent per ounce on drinks with added caloric sweetener; exempts 100% juice, artificially sweetened beverages, infant formula, milk products, medical drinks, and alcoholic beverages. Implemented April 2017

BERKELEY, CA: 1 cent per ounce on sweetened drinks; exempts meal-replacement and dairy drinks, diet sodas, 100% fruit juice, and alcohol. Implemented March 2015

OAKLAND, CA: 1 cent per ounce on drinks with added sugars; exempts 100% juice, artificially sweetened beverages, infant formula, milk products, medical drinks, and alcoholic beverages. Implemented July 2017

MEXICO: 1 peso per liter ($0.05) on all drinks with added sugar, excluding milks or yogurts. Implemented January 2014

COLOMBIA: VAT on soft drinks now applied as multiphase tax at production, distribution, and commercialization phases of supply chain (previously VAT only applied to production phase). Implemented January 1, 2019

PERU: 25% tax (increase from 17%) on non-alcoholic beverages with ≥6 g sugar per 100 ml; drinks with <6 g sugar per 100 ml, including bottled waters, remain at 17% tax rate. Implemented May 2018

BOULDER, CO: 2 cents per ounce on beverages with added sugars or sweeteners. Implemented July 2017

PHILADELPHIA, PA: 1.5 cents per ounce on sugar- and artificially-sweetened drinks, including diet soda. Implemented January 2017

NAVAJO NATION: 2% junk food tax on "minimal-to-no nutritional value food items," including SSBs. Implemented April 2015

BERMUDA: 50% import tax on sugar, sugary drinks, candies and dilutables; exempts diet sodas, 100% juice, and diet iced teas. Implemented October 2018 Increases to 75% import tax Implemented April 2019

BARBADOS: 10% excise tax on sugary drinks, including carbonated soft drinks, juice drinks, and sports drinks; exempts 100% juice, coconut water, and plain milk. Implemented August 2015

DOMINICA: 10% excise tax on food and drinks with high sugar content, including soft drinks and energy drinks. Implemented September 2015

CHILE: 18% ad valorem tax on sugary drinks containing >6.25 g sugar per 100 ml includes all non-alcoholic drinks with added sweeteners; exempts 100% fruit juice and dairy-based beverages; 10% ad valorem tax on drinks with <6.25 g sugar per 100 ml. Implemented October 2014

■ Implemented   ■ Passed

Source: Global Food Research Program, University of North Carolina, http://globalfoodresearchprogram.web.unc.edu/multi-country-initiative /resources/.

Note: The map was created based on the dataset available as of March 2019. g = gram; ml = milliliter; VAT = value added tax.

Map 5.3 Sugar-Sweetened Beverage Taxes: Europe and Northern Africa

IBRD 44266 | DECEMBER 2019

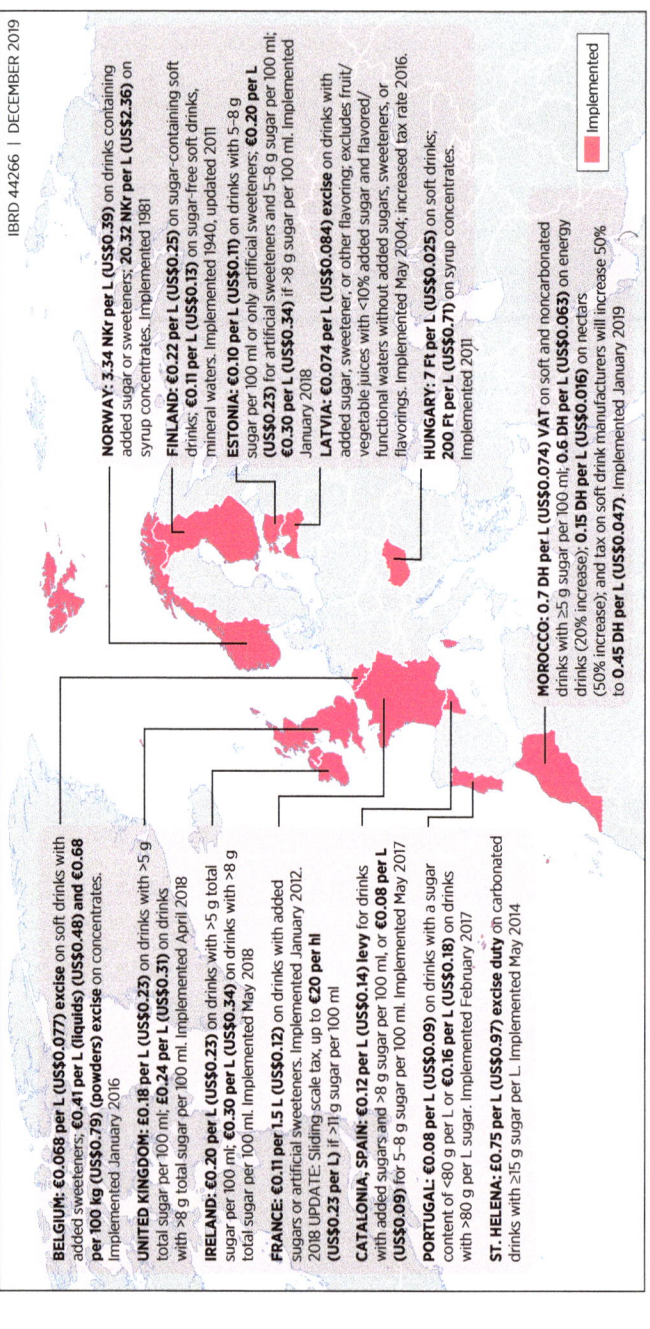

NORWAY: 3.34 NKr per L (US$0.39) on drinks containing added sugar or sweeteners; **20.32 NKr per L (US$2.36)** on syrup concentrates. Implemented 1981

FINLAND: €0.22 per L (US$0.25) on sugar-containing soft drinks; **€0.11 per L (US$0.13)** on sugar-free soft drinks, mineral waters. Implemented 1940, updated 2011

ESTONIA: €0.10 per L (US$0.11) on drinks with 5–8 g sugar per 100 ml or only artificial sweeteners; **€0.20 per L (US$0.23)** for artificial sweeteners and 5–8 g sugar per 100 ml; **€0.30 per L (US$0.34)** if >8 g sugar per 100 ml. Implemented January 2018

LATVIA: €0.074 per L (US$0.084) excise on drinks with added sugar, sweetener, or other flavoring; excludes fruit/vegetable juices with <10% added sugars and flavored/functional waters without added sugars, sweeteners, or flavorings. Implemented May 2004; increased tax rate 2016.

HUNGARY: 7 Ft per L (US$0.025) on soft drinks; **200 Ft per L (US$0.71)** on syrup concentrates. Implemented 2011

MOROCCO: 0.7 DH per L (US$0.074) VAT on soft and noncarbonated drinks with ≥5 g sugar per 100 ml; **0.6 DH per L (US$0.063)** on energy drinks (20% increase); **0.15 DH per L (US$0.016)** on nectars (50% increase); and tax on soft drink manufacturers will increase 50% to **0.45 DH per L (US$0.047)**. Implemented January 2019

BELGIUM: €0.068 per L (US$0.077) excise on soft drinks with added sweeteners; **€0.41 per L (liquids) (US$0.48)** and **€0.68 per 100 kg (US$0.79) (powders) excise** on concentrates. Implemented January 2016

UNITED KINGDOM: £0.18 per L (US$0.23) on drinks with >5 g total sugar per 100 ml; **£0.24 per L (US$0.31)** on drinks with >8 g total sugar per 100 ml. Implemented April 2018

IRELAND: €0.20 per L (US$0.23) on drinks with >5 g total sugar per 100 ml; **€0.30 per L (US$0.34)** on drinks with >8 g total sugar per 100 ml. Implemented May 2018

FRANCE: €0.11 per 1.5 L (US$0.12) on drinks with added sugars or artificial sweeteners. Implemented January 2012. 2018 UPDATE: Sliding scale tax, up to **€20 per hl (US$0.23 per L)** if >11 g sugar per 100 ml

CATALONIA, SPAIN: €0.12 per L (US$0.14) levy for drinks with added sugars and >8 g sugar per 100 ml, or **€0.08 per L (US$0.09)** for 5–8 g sugar per 100 ml. Implemented May 2017

PORTUGAL: €0.08 per L (US$0.09) on drinks with a sugar content of <80 g per L or **€0.16 per L (US$0.18)** on drinks with >80 g per L sugar. Implemented February 2017

ST. HELENA: £0.75 per L (US$0.97) excise duty on carbonated drinks with ≥15 g sugar per L. Implemented May 2014

Implemented

Source: Global Food Research Program, University of North Carolina, http://globalfoodresearchprogram.web.unc.edu/multi-country-initiative/resources/.

Note: The map was created based on the dataset available as of March 2019. g = gram; hl = hectoliter; kg = kilogram; L = liter; ml = milliliter.

Map 5.4 Sugar-Sweetened Beverage Taxes: Sub-Saharan Africa, Asia, and the Pacific

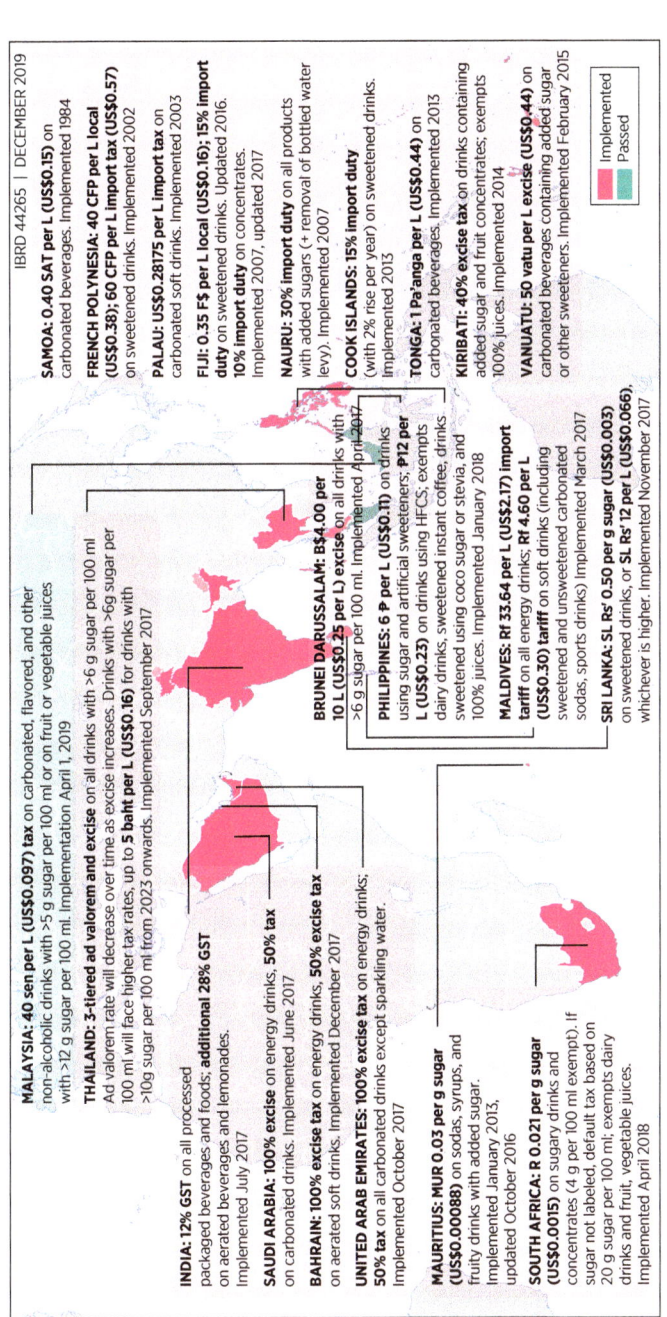

IBRD 44265 | DECEMBER 2019

MALAYSIA: 40 sen per L (US$0.097) tax on carbonated, flavored, and other non-alcoholic drinks with >5 g sugar per 100 ml or on fruit or vegetable juices with >12 g sugar per 100 ml. Implemented April 1, 2019

THAILAND: 3-tiered ad valorem and excise on all drinks with >6 g sugar per 100 ml. Ad valorem rate will decrease over time as excise increases. Drinks with >6g sugar per 100 ml will face higher tax rates, up to **5 baht per L (US$0.16)** for drinks with >10g sugar per 100 ml from 2023 onwards. Implemented September 2017

INDIA: 12% GST on all processed packaged beverages and foods; **additional 28% GST** on aerated beverages and lemonades. Implemented July 2017

SAUDI ARABIA: 100% excise on energy drinks, **50% tax** on carbonated drinks. Implemented June 2017

BAHRAIN: 100% excise tax on energy drinks, **50% excise tax** on aerated soft drinks. Implemented December 2017

UNITED ARAB EMIRATES: 100% excise tax on energy drinks; **50% tax** on all carbonated drinks except sparkling water. Implemented October 2017

MAURITIUS: MUR 0.03 per g sugar (US$0.00088) on sodas, syrups, and fruity drinks with added sugar. Implemented January 2013, updated October 2016

SOUTH AFRICA: R 0.021 per g sugar (US$0.0015) on sugary drinks and concentrates (4 g per 100 ml exempt). If sugar not labeled, default tax based on 20 g sugar per 100 ml; exempts dairy drinks and fruit, vegetable juices. Implemented April 2018

BRUNEI DARUSSALAM: B$4.00 per 10 L (US$0.25 per L) excise on all drinks with >6 g sugar per 100 ml. Implemented April 2017

PHILIPPINES: 6 ₱ per L (US$0.11) on drinks using sugar and artificial sweeteners; **₱12 per L (US$0.23)** on drinks using HFCS; exempts dairy drinks, sweetened instant coffee, drinks sweetened using coco sugar or stevia, and 100% juices. Implemented January 2018

MALDIVES: Rf 33.64 per L (US$2.17) import tariff on all energy drinks; **Rf 4.60 per L (US$0.30) tariff** on soft drinks (including sweetened and unsweetened carbonated sodas, sports drinks) Implemented March 2017

SRI LANKA: SLRs' 0.50 per g sugar (US$0.003) on sweetened drinks, or **SL Rs'12 per L (US$0.066)**, whichever is higher. Implemented November 2017

SAMOA: 0.40 SAT per L (US$0.15) on carbonated beverages. Implemented 1984

FRENCH POLYNESIA: 40 CFP per L local (US$0.38); 60 CFP per L import tax (US$0.57) on sweetened drinks. Implemented 2002

PALAU: US$0.28175 per L import tax on carbonated soft drinks. Implemented 2003

FIJI: 0.35 F$ per L local (US$0.16); 15% import duty on sweetened drinks. Updated 2016. **10% import duty** on concentrates. Implemented 2007, updated 2017

NAURU: 30% import duty on all products with added sugars (+ removal of bottled water levy). Implemented 2007

COOK ISLANDS: 15% import duty (with 2% rise per year) on sweetened drinks. Implemented 2013

TONGA: 1 Pa'anga per L (US$0.44) on carbonated beverages. Implemented 2013

KIRIBATI: 40% excise tax on drinks containing added sugar and fruit concentrates; exempts 100% juices. Implemented 2014

VANUATU: 50 vatu per L excise (US$0.44) on carbonated beverages containing added sugar or other sweeteners. Implemented February 2015

☐ Implemented
☐ Passed

Source: Global Food Research Program, University of North Carolina, http://globalfoodresearchprogram.web.unc.edu/multi-country-initiative /resources/.

Note: The map was created based on the dataset available as of March 2019. g = gram; GST = goods and services tax; HFCS = high-fructose corn syrup; L = liter; ml = milliliter.

be exempt from VAT to prevent hardship on low-income households. Subsidies and tax exemptions mainly benefit households with high consumption of the targeted product and the poor who are more sensitive to price changes; thus, policy to reduce prices mainly works as an income transfer policy and, to a lesser extent, as a nutritional intervention (Chakrabarti, Kishore, and Roy 2018; de Walque 2018).

Diet-related taxes are mainly levied on SSBs and foods high in added saturated fat, sodium, or sugar—often termed junk foods, nonessential foods, or ultra-processed foods. The advantages of taxing SSBs are linked both to the impact of sugar on health and to the inability of the body to compensate for the calories from a beverage by reducing food intake (DiMeglio and Mattes 2000; Mourao et al. 2007; WCRFI 2015; WHO 2014).

Taxation for Sugar-Sweetened Beverages: Design, Impact, and Challenges

Taxing SSBs successfully requires careful consideration of the design of the tax in the context of the specific country involved and an understanding of both its expected impact including substitution patterns and the challenges inherent in such a policy.

Design of SSB Taxes

The design of a diet-related tax needs to consider the objectives set by a government and economic realities related to the market structures of unhealthy products. Design issues include whether diet-related taxes are structured as a specific excise tax based on the "unhealthy" content in a product or as an ad valorem tax based on a percentage of the price. A specific excise tax is a per unit tax—for example, a tax based on the sugar or fat content of a product or the product volume, such as one pound of sugar. These excise taxes can be tiered, as with the U.K. and South African systems where low sugar content is untaxed and the rates change with the amount of sugar used in the product. Excise taxes on content can have a greater impact on consumers who switch to healthier alternatives than those who do not, as well as on producers who have an incentive to reduce unhealthy content such as sugar (Briggs et al. 2017). These taxes are also better targeted, because the product price increases with a greater unhealthy content. Because a tax on content is independent from the product price, it will prevent consumers from switching from more expensive to lower-priced products. Still, some countries combine their excise tax with an ad valorem tax as a percentage of the retail price of the product.

More recently governments have begun to consider taxes that would affect supply and demand, with reformulation of the content to create healthier beverages and foods being the prime supply goal. Two countries— South Africa and the United Kingdom—were the first, in 2018, to initiate such taxes. In April 2018, South Africa introduced a health promotion levy that left untaxed items with less than 4 grams of sugar per 100 milliliters and then taxed the grams of sugar in products. The tax is 2.1 cents per gram for beverages with a sugar content exceeding 4 grams per 100 milliliters, which translates into about 11 percent of the retail price (National Treasury 2016).[1] A slightly more complex version of this tax is the tax the United Kingdom introduced with its Soft Drink Industry Levy in August 2018, which directly targets producers and importers of sugary soft drinks. The goal of the levy is to encourage manufacturers to produce healthier products, remove added sugar, reduce portion sizes, and promote diet beverages. Soft drink companies are charged on beverages with added sugar and total sugar content of 4 grams or more per 100 milliliters, or about 4 percent sugar content. The levy is higher for beverages containing 8 grams or more per 100 milliliters, in which case the sugar levy is 18 pence a liter or 24 pence a liter if the sugar content is over 8 grams per 100 milliliters.

The question that remains unresolved as it relates to these tiered and nutrient-related taxes is whether promoting reformulation, which typically involves a rapid increase in diet sweeteners—primarily in high-income countries—is healthful. At this point, the global consensus has been to support reformulation but several countries are considering labeling foods and beverages containing diet sweeteners with that information on the front-of-package label (for example, "contains diet sweeteners").

Fiscal Policy and SSB Taxes: The Evidence of Impact to Date

Taxation policy often spurs debate on equity and efficiency objectives. Efficient taxation curbs unhealthy consumption without negatively affecting individual welfare as a result of higher prices (Härkänen et al. 2014). It has been argued that diet-related taxes levied on unhealthy products can increase efficiency because they aim to influence unhealthy consumption and subsequently curb the incidence of costly diseases. Taxes on consumption—including diet-related taxes—are considered inequitable if the poor spend a higher proportion of their income than the rich on taxed goods.

On the other hand, taxes have a pro-poor welfare effect if the poor are more sensitive to price changes and subsequently reduce their intake of unhealthy products. As a result, the poor would benefit disproportionately more than the rich from the health benefits of adjusted consumption.

This is the subpopulation most likely to have undiagnosed, untreated, or poorly treated non-communicable diseases linked to excessive SSB intakes. It can therefore be argued that a diet-related tax is expected to increase the overall welfare of consumers since it will reduce unhealthy consumption, particularly for low-income groups, and curb related societal costs. The tax also becomes pro-poor if it is used to finance public services such as health care predominantly used by the poor (Begg, Fischer, and Dornbusch 2000), as discussed in an earlier chapter.

Over 42 countries have instituted SSB taxes. Many are smaller Pacific or Caribbean Island countries with high overweight/obesity rates, but a number of large countries have also introduced SSB taxes. To date, most of the taxes have been based on the volume of drinks consumed and tax at the distributor/manufacturer level, not on the sugar content of the product—this is the case in the United Kingdom and South Africa, discussed earlier. Sin taxes on tobacco and alcohol have a long history; the World Health Organization (WHO) and the broader health community anticipated that SSB taxes would work equally well, but the particular substitutions that would take place had to be studied to understand the net effect (Brownell et al. 2009; WHO Commission on Ending Childhood Obesity 2016).

One critical question for any caloric beverage- or food-related tax is its impact and the potential for substitution. Most evaluations use food purchase data sets that are usually representative of the urban segment of each country. Mexico's SSB tax, its price pass-through, and its impact are discussed in box 5.1. In that case, water was found to be the major substitute. Taxes based on volume have generally followed a pattern similar to the experience in Mexico. Volume-based taxes in Barbados, Chile, France, and in Berkeley, California and Philadelphia, Pennsylvania in the United States for example, have reduced SSB purchase slightly less than a higher tax rate would suggest. Chile increased the tax on most SSBs from 13 percent to 18 percent while reducing the tax rate from 13 percent to 10 percent on diet beverages and concentrates (a key SSB substitute for the poor). Price increases in the 3.1–3.5 percent range were found by two studies using identical data; however, one found purchases declined slightly, which seemed appropriate for this small price increase (a volume reduction of 3.4 percent in SSBs, an increase in low-taxed items of 10.7 percent, and a total calorie decrease of 4.0 percent; Caro et al. 2018). A different study with the same data found the unbelievable result of a 21.6 percent decline in the volume of higher taxed SSBs purchased, with no effect on the lower tax category in Chile (Nakamura et al. 2018). These two studies are indicative of the complexity of studying the impact of these complex taxes using different econometric approaches and classifying products into various tax categories.

The Impact of Taxes on Sugar-Sweetened Beverages and Nonessential Foods in Mexico

Mexico's prevalence of overweight/obesity and diabetes is one of the highest in the world. This burden falls disproportionately on lower-income Mexicans, who also are most likely to have undiagnosed or poorly treated diabetes. To address these issues, the Mexican government implemented a peso-per-liter tax on sugar-sweetened beverages (SSBs) and an 8 percent tax on nonessential foods with energy density ≥ 275 kilocalories per 100 grams. These were the first taxes in either category to be rigorously evaluated with representative food purchase data.

Price pass-through results in the first year showed that the SSB tax was passed through at greater than its approximate pretax 10 percent level on small sizes of beverages and in urban areas relative to larger-sized containers and poorer rural areas (Colchero, Salgado, Unar-Munguía, Molina, et al. 2015; Colchero, Zavala et al. 2017).

The impact of this tax in the first year was an approximate 6 percent overall decline in purchases followed by an additional 4 percent decline in the second year (Colchero et al. 2016; Colchero, Rivera-Dommarco et al. 2017). To estimate these effects, the researchers estimated changes in household purchases of beverages in 2014 compared with 2012 and 2013 (see figure B5.1.1). Longitudinal fixed effects models that examined the difference in trends before and after the tax (difference-in-differences model) were to account for a preexisting decline in SSB purchases over the two-year period prior to the tax. Household socioeconomic status and composition along with contextual controls for changing economic conditions (city-level unemployment and salary levels) were used.

In the first year, the tax had the greatest impact among lower socioeconomic households, with a 9 percent average decline in purchases of sugary drinks over 2014 and a 17 percent decline by December 2014 (see figure B5.1.2). The top socioeconomic status tertile did not significantly reduce SSB purchases. Furthermore, the purchase of untaxed beverages increased by 4 percent overall, primarily driven by an increase in bottled water purchases. This meant about 12.8 liters of additional water purchased. Figure B5.1.3 highlights the additional impact of the tax in the second year. Additional research found that the largest consumers reduced their intake the most. Groups that typically had high purchases of the taxed beverages saw the largest

continued next page

Box 5.1 (*continued*)

Figure B5.1.1   Impact of Sugar-Sweetened Beverage Taxes in Mexico in Year 1

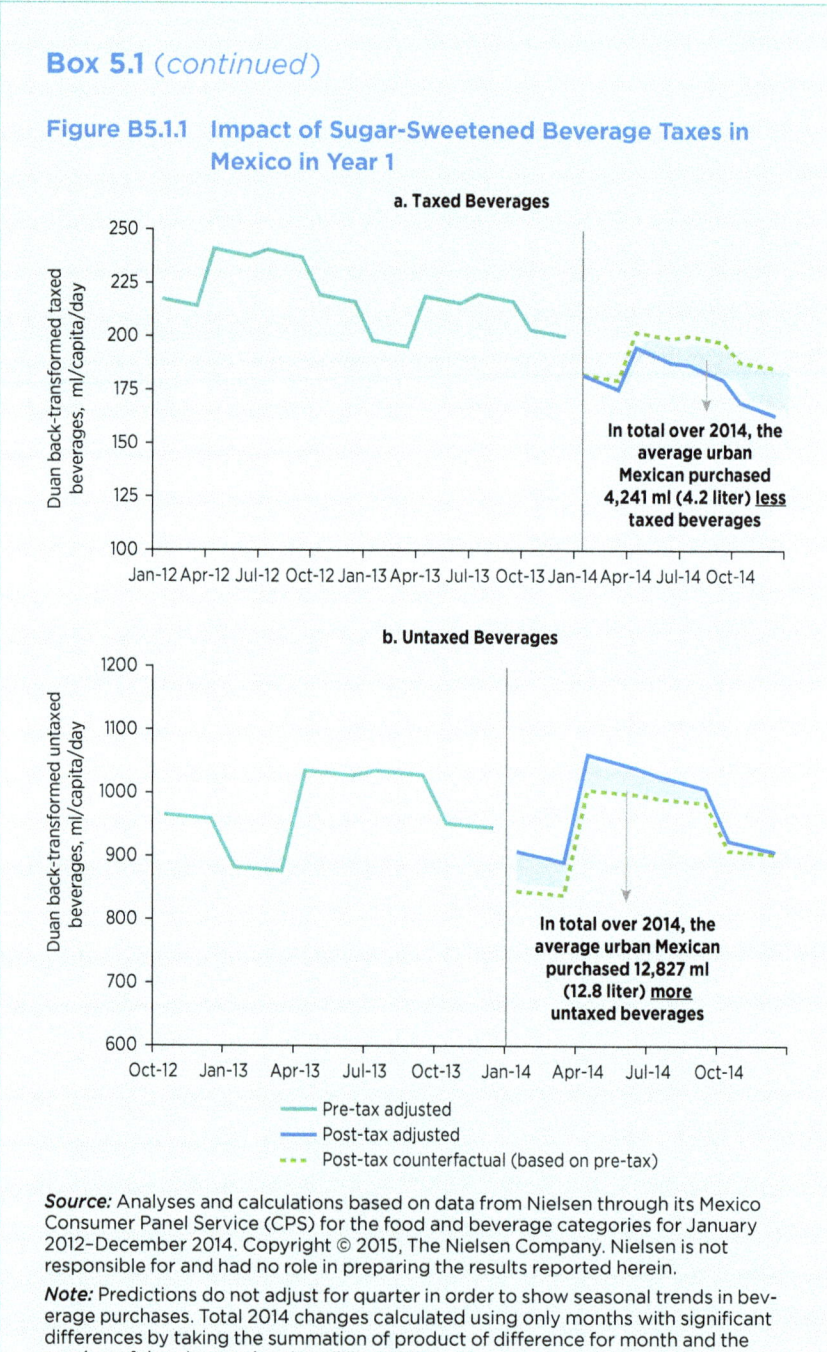

a. Taxed Beverages

In total over 2014, the average urban Mexican purchased 4,241 ml (4.2 liter) <u>less</u> taxed beverages

b. Untaxed Beverages

In total over 2014, the average urban Mexican purchased 12,827 ml (12.8 liter) <u>more</u> untaxed beverages

Pre-tax adjusted
Post-tax adjusted
Post-tax counterfactual (based on pre-tax)

Source: Analyses and calculations based on data from Nielsen through its Mexico Consumer Panel Service (CPS) for the food and beverage categories for January 2012–December 2014. Copyright © 2015, The Nielsen Company. Nielsen is not responsible for and had no role in preparing the results reported herein.

Note: Predictions do not adjust for quarter in order to show seasonal trends in beverage purchases. Total 2014 changes calculated using only months with significant differences by taking the summation of product of difference for month and the number of days in month. ml = milliliter; SSB = sugar-sweetened beverage.

continued next page

Box 5.1 (continued)

Figure B5.1.2 Impact of Sugar-Sweetened Beverage Tax in Mexico in Year 1 by Socioeconomic Status (SES)

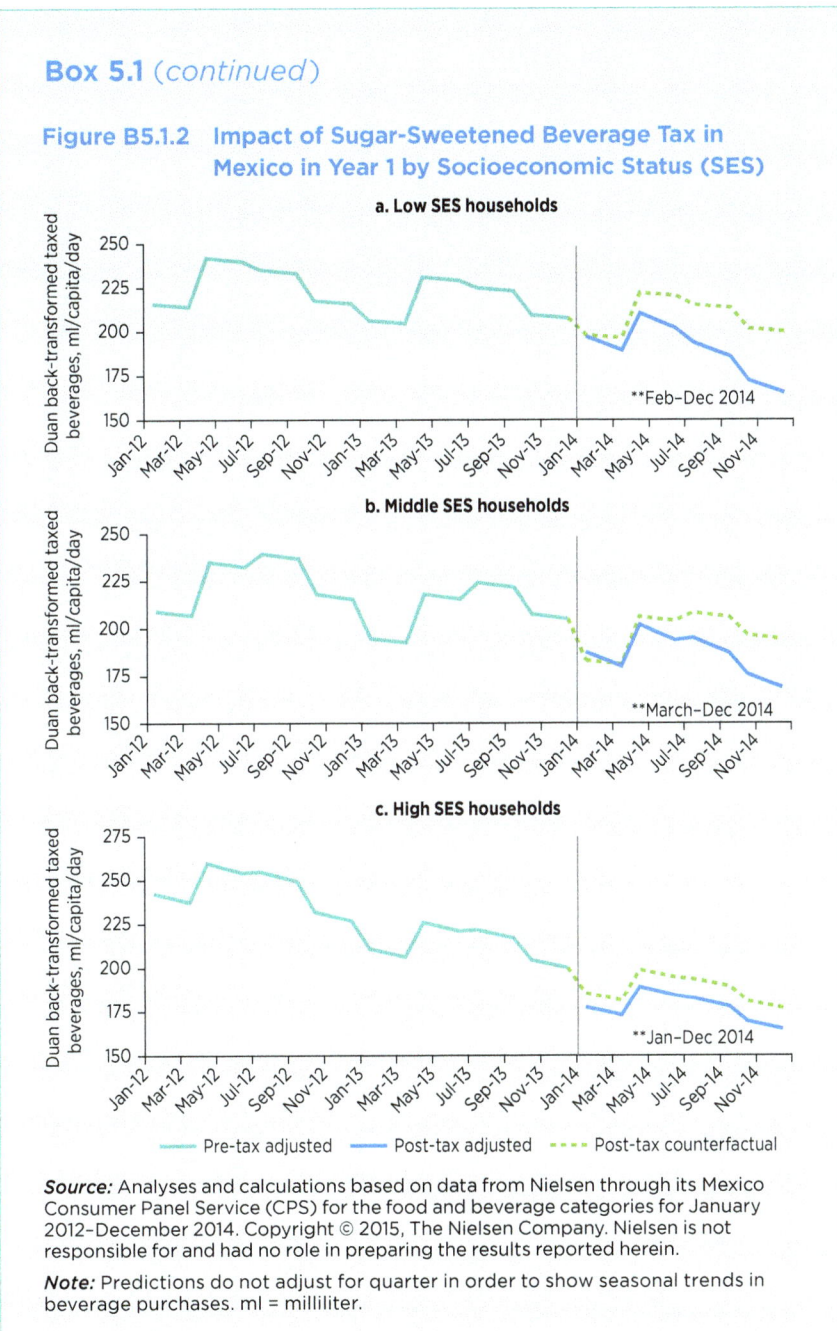

a. Low SES households

b. Middle SES households

c. High SES households

Pre-tax adjusted — Post-tax adjusted — Post-tax counterfactual

Source: Analyses and calculations based on data from Nielsen through its Mexico Consumer Panel Service (CPS) for the food and beverage categories for January 2012–December 2014. Copyright © 2015, The Nielsen Company. Nielsen is not responsible for and had no role in preparing the results reported herein.

Note: Predictions do not adjust for quarter in order to show seasonal trends in beverage purchases. ml = milliliter.

continued next page

Box 5.1 (*continued*)

Figure B5.1.3   Two-Year Impact of Sugar-Sweetened Beverage Tax in Mexico

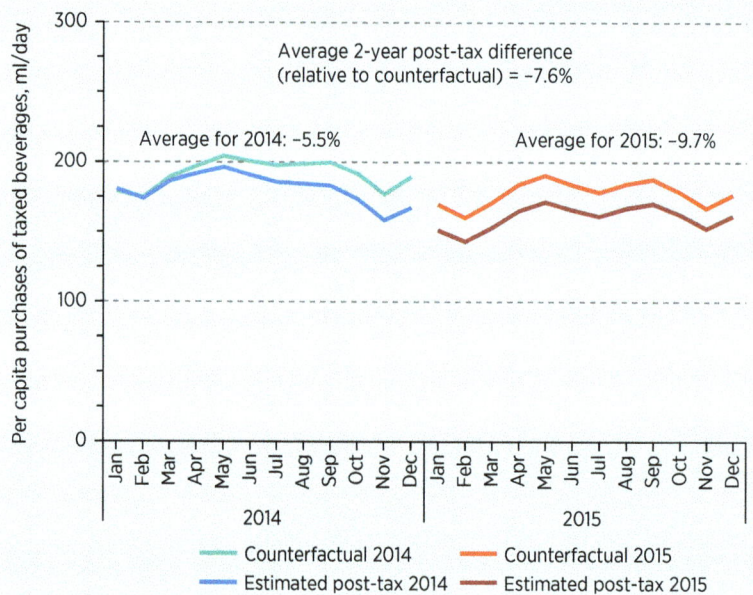

Source: Colchero, Rivera-Dommarco et al. 2017.

Note: ml = milliliter; SSB = sugar-sweetened beverage.

reduction (–18 percent) in those purchases, as well as the largest increase (+12 percent) in purchases of untaxed beverages by 2015, the second year of the tax (Ng et al. 2018).

The nonessential food tax followed the same methodology as the SSB tax (Batis et al. 2016; Taillie et al. 2017). The post-tax declines in

continued next page

Box 5.1 *(continued)*

the percentage of taxed food purchases increased from 4.8 percent in the first year to 7.4 percent in the second year, yielding a two-year mean decline of 6.0 percent beyond the counterfactual (p<0.01). Post-tax change in the percentage of taxed food purchases varied by pre-tax purchasing level. Most importantly, the major change was found in those who were unhealthy food purchasers before the tax. The positive effect of Mexico's junk food tax continued in the second year, and households with greater earlier preferences for taxed foods showed a larger decline in taxed food purchases.

Employment research found that there were no reductions in the number of employees either in the SSB or energy-dense food manufacturing industries or in the Mexican commercial establishments after the taxes were implemented (Guerrero-López, Molina, and Colchero 2017).

Barbados introduced a 10 percent ad valorem tax on SSBs but omitted taxing powdered drinks (a major substitute). Using point-of-sale data from the major chain on the island, the authors found sales of SSBs decreased by 4.3 percent. Sales of non-SSBs increased by 5.2 percent, with water sales increasing an average of 7.5 percent (Alvarado et al. 2019).

The government of France introduced an SSB tax of €0.072 per liter (more recently increased, albeit without an evaluation, to a higher tax with a sliding scale tax of up to €20 per hectoliter [US$0.23 per liter] if there are more than 11 grams of sugar per 100 milliliters). Based on a study of about a half million price records for non-alcoholic beverages, the tax was shifted to cover all carbonated beverages and partially to fruit drinks (Berardi et al. 2016). An alternate study in France compared consumer purchase data from two French regions and two neighboring Italian regions with longitudinal fixed effects models and found differential price increases linked to the tax by drink category with an average of €0.07–€0.08 (Capacci et al. 2016). They also found a statistically significant but small reduction in purchases of carbonated SSBs (0.08 liters per week) and fruit drinks (0.4 liters per week) and an overall decline in taxed drinks (of 0.09 liters per week).

A variety of U.S. cities have instituted taxes. The most important set of evaluations to date are for Philadelphia, a large city with a large poor population, which put in place a tax of 1.5 cents per U.S.

ounce (approximately 15 percent). Preliminary results have been published online by several groups (Cawley et al. 2018; Seiler, Tuchman, and Yao 2019). Enormous variance in methods and results have occurred, but generally most studies find purchases dropped significantly, reducing the frequency of SSB consumption by over 10 times per month (Cawley et al. 2018). Price pass-through varied greatly by type of retailer, with a net reduction of sales estimated at 38 percent after reconsidering leakage to other areas and sales trends (Roberto et al. 2019). The only other publications to date relate to the small city of Berkeley where initial consumption was very low; nevertheless, the tax affected prices and reduced SSB purchases. An array of publications using sales data (Silver et al. 2017) or consumer intercept data (Falbe et al. 2015; Falbe et al. 2016) have found the tax impact on prices to be fairly complex, with price changes equal to the tax in major retail outlets but no increases in small convenience stores; nevertheless, SSB purchases declined overall. Overall, the higher decline found in Philadelphia could reflect the higher tax, much greater initial consumption, or a poorer population. All of these issues are impactful.

SSBs have been the major taxation target for two clear reasons. First, consuming a beverage does not impact food intake. Second, sugar has unique adverse health effects. A systematic review of 30 publications from 1996 to 2005 found a positive association between greater intakes of SSBs (particularly soda) and weight gain and overweight/obesity in both children and adults (Malik and Hu 2015). Another meta-analysis considering 88 studies found clear associations of soft drink intake with increased energy intake and body weight. SSB consumption was also linked to lower intakes of milk as well as calcium and other nutrients and to an increased risk of several health problems, including diabetes (Vartanian, Schwartz, and Brownell 2007). A sophisticated set of studies on the health impacts of the Mexican SSB tax estimated that it would result in about 189,300 fewer incident type 2 diabetes cases, 20,400 fewer incident strokes and myocardial infarctions, and 18,900 fewer deaths occurring from 2013 to 2022 (Sánchez-Romero et al. 2016); a second estimated that by 2030, the tax would reduce obesity by 2.5 percent (Barrientos-Gutierrez et al. 2017).

The major issues about tax design remain unsettled until more evaluations are put in place, including evaluations of the two nutrient-based taxes. These are the three-tiered U.K. tax rate system based on grams of sugar levied at the manufacturer level and the South African per gram of sugar tax system. Very high tax rates—such as the 50 percent SSB taxes in Saudi Arabia and the United Arab Emirates—have also not been evaluated as yet.

Challenges

Any diet-related tax will face challenges. The main challenges to their successful implementation are a tax system's administrative capacity, substitution effects, tax evasion, and opposition from the food industry. These challenges need to be considered when designing effective tax policies. A useful guide to many of the issues to consider was published by the World Cancer Research Fund (WCRFI 2015).

Successful implementation of any tax will depend on, among other things, the effectiveness of tax administration. Countries with strong tax administrations generally design excise taxes based on nutrient content. Alternatively, taxes on product volumes may be easier to implement in countries where tax administration is not so strong. It is generally easier for tax administrators to collect and enforce taxes if they are levied on the producer or wholesalers, as there are fewer producers and wholesalers than retailers that would have to comply with the tax (IMF 2016). For taxes based on nutrient levels such as grams of sugar, countries have employed defaults to the highest tax level when the product lacked adequate nutrition facts front-of-package labeling data; this is a very effective method of getting nutrition facts front-of-package labeling data added.

The substitution effect posits that consumers will switch to lower-priced products. It limits the impact of a sugar tax on total sugar consumption if consumers who like sugar find a substitute for sugary beverages and will drink, for example, more fruit juices (Fletcher 2011). The Mexican and Chilean experiences did not find this. Instead, in Mexico consumers substituted bottled water for SSBs after the SSB tax went into effect; and in Chile there were no signs of increasing purchase of additional kilocalories of other beverages (Caro et al. 2018; Colchero et al. 2016). The experience from the United States with soda taxes shows that consumers—children and teenagers especially—may switch to other high-calorie drinks that are relatively inexpensive, meaning there is little or no effect on excess weight and obesity (Fletcher, Frisvold, and Tefft 2013). If individuals switch from sugary drinks to foods that are even higher in calories or high in fat and sodium, then the calorie intake could even increase and diminish any health gains that may be achieved through reduced sugar intake. However, findings from the United States suggest that substitution to other beverages mainly involved fruit juices, and there was no evidence of substitution with sugary foods and no effect on total sodium purchased (Finkelstein et al. 2013). To date, most countries planning such sin taxes in the food area have first used demand systems to study food and beverage substitutes and found most substitutes to be healthful (Caro, Ng, Bonilla et al. 2017; Caro, Ng, Taillie et al. 2017; Colchero, Salgado, Unar-Munguía, Hernández-Ávila, and Rivera-Dommarco 2015; Colchero, Salgado, Unar-Munguía, Molina et al. 2015; Stacey, Tugendhaft, and Hofman 2017).

Another challenge is that consumers may try to avoid paying diet-related taxes through cross-border purchases. The short-lived saturated fat tax in Denmark, for example, led Danes to purchase non-taxed products across the border in Germany or Sweden (Smed et al. 2016). Similarly, it is estimated that about 10 percent of the alcohol market in the United Kingdom and 20 percent of the cigarette market in France take place across the border. Such cross-border purchases can limit the effectiveness of taxes. Setting tax rates therefore requires an understanding of the purchasing behavior of consumers, of tax rates in neighboring markets, and of the effectiveness of the tax authority to enforce compliance. A regional approach to taxation can reduce the evasion effect. At the same time, leakage into purchases from other countries is less likely for a product as bulky as SSBs but much more likely for cigarettes and ultra-processed foods.

The highly concentrated food and beverage industry constantly challenges diet-related taxes. The beverage and food markets consist of few manufacturers sharing a large share of total production. In France, for example, the top two soft drink manufacturers share 89 percent of total production (Bonnet and Réquillart 2013). Because of this concentrated market situation, the food and beverage industry will challenge diet-related taxes through aggressive marketing campaigns for sugary drinks and highly processed foods. In 2014, the beverage industry in California spent more than US$10 million on advertising campaigns to fight sugar taxes on beverages (WHO Expert Committee 2016). In Philadelphia, the soft drink industry pledged to donate US$10 million to the Children's Hospital of Philadelphia if the city council voted down the sugar tax.[2] In 2018, the American beverage industry had its appeal to the Pennsylvania Supreme Court granted; it unsuccessfully challenged the legality of Philadelphia's sugar tax (Du et al. 2018). These examples show that industry interests are powerful and could influence the lifespan of a tax. The *New York Times* documented similar efforts in Colombia, Mexico, and a number of other countries in which not only did the food industry engage in counter-marketing activities but it also used much more personal attacks against advocacy leaders and scholars supporting taxes and other regulations; additionally, it utilized trade negotiations and other legal approaches (Jacobs and Richtel 2017a, 2017b). Despite these industry attacks, for fiscal and health reasons an increasing number of countries (as shown in maps 5.2, 5.3, and 5.4) are introducing SSB taxes.

The following section presents experiences from selected countries, including how they have designed and implemented diet-related taxes and the challenges they have faced. Thereafter, the final section presents lessons and recommendations for countries interested in diet-related taxes.

Diet-Related Taxation

Diet-related taxes have been introduced in Finland, France, and Hungary in 2011; followed by Chile, Mexico, and Mauritius in 2014; and, most recently, in the Gulf Cooperation Council countries, South Africa, and Thailand. The highest diet-related taxes are levied in Saudi Arabia and the United Arab Emirates, where they amount to 50 percent of the price of soda and 100 percent of the price of energy drinks. It is important to note that none of these taxes have focused directly on ultra-processed foods, but recent studies of the health impact of these foods suggest that this is a critical future direction to consider (Hall 2019; Rico-Campà et al. 2019; Srour et al. 2019).

Design of Diet-Related Taxes

To examine countries' experience with taxes, the World Bank conducted nine case studies on dietary policies in Brazil, Chile, Mexico, Poland, South Africa, Sri Lanka, Thailand, Turkey, and the state of Kerala in India. Chile has the highest consumption of sugary beverages in the world (Popkin and Hawkes 2015), a very high junk food intake, and high overweight/obesity prevalence (Cediel et al. 2017; Corvalán et al. 2018; Popkin and Reardon 2018). High levels of SSB consumption, combined with high overweight/ obesity rates and increasing prevalence of related diseases, have prompted the introduction of diet-related taxes in five of the nine cases studied (table 5.2 presents an overview). Governments argued that taxes would lead to higher prices and, combined with other public health measures, would cause consumers to reduce their sugar intake, which would help reduce their weight and improve their health status. The five case study areas that introduced diet-related taxes were focused on taxing beverages with high sugar content. Of this group, only Mexico also taxes unhealthy foods (Batis et al. 2016). Kerala's fat tax on unhealthy food was abolished after one year.

When designing a diet-related tax, governments make decisions about which products to tax based on content or volume or price, and whether the tax will be a specific excise or an ad valorem tax on the price. As noted earlier, the first product considered for taxation linked to public health has been SSBs. In September 2014, Chile increased the tax rate from 13 percent to 18 percent for SSBs that have a sugar content higher than 15 grams per 240 milliliters or equivalent portion. The rate was reduced to 10 percent for other beverages (Caro et al. 2018). In 2018, South Africa introduced a sugar levy of 2.1 cents per gram for beverages with a sugar content exceeding 4 grams per 100 milliliters, which translates into about 11 percent of the retail price. This is the first low- or middle-income country that has used a nutrient-based tax for SSBs.

In Thailand, beverage retailers are also taxed based on the amount of sugar in their SSBs (table 5.2). The new excise tax rates in the country are not expected to lead to a significant increase in the prices of sugar-sweetened carbonated drinks, whereas the SSB tax will lead to higher prices for sugar-sweetened tea, coffee, and fruit and vegetable drinks with excess sugar. Prices are likely to increase: for example, a 500 milliliter bottle of tea that contains 54.5 grams of sugar will be taxed at 10 percent per value and 0.5 baht (US$0.015) per liter. This tax is quite complex and its rate increases over time, with the government's goal being to encourage reformulation. The sugar tax increases every two years; by 2023 onward the tax will be approximately 1 baht (US$0.03) per liter for drinks containing 6–8 grams, 3 baht (around US$0.095) for drinks containing from 8 to 10 grams, and 5 baht (around US$0.15) per liter for drinks with over 10 grams.

Mexico taxes unhealthy food and beverages, whereas other countries mainly tax beverages high in sugar content. Kerala also had a fat tax on unhealthy foods, but it was in effect for only a year. The fat tax in Kerala was an ad valorem tax of 14.5 percent of the price levied on burgers, pizzas, tacos, doughnuts, sandwiches, pasta, and bread fillings sold by restaurants with an international brand name or trade mark registration. This made international restaurant chains such as Kentucky Fried Chicken, Pizza Hut, Dominos, Chic King, French Fried Chicken, Southern Fried Chicken, and McDonald's the primary targets of the tax. As such, the fat tax was based on the type of food business operator and not the content of unhealthy product. The Kerala government planned to start with branded products and slowly expand the fat tax to unhealthy food items sold by bakeries and other local eateries. From the start this tax addressed only international fast food chains and missed the bulk of unhealthy fast food consumption from local stalls and chains.

An excise tax based on volume is more practical to implement than an ad valorem tax. Mexico and Thailand introduced a combination of excise and ad valorem taxes. A specific excise per gram of sugar content instead of liter or kilogram will result in higher taxes for products higher in sugar content. However, sugar excise taxes in Mexico are per liter of beverage, which results in a lower tax per gram of sugar content for more sugary drinks (Colchero et al. 2016; Colchero, Salgado, Unar-Munguía, Hernández-Ávila, and Rivera-Dommarco 2015).

Diet-related taxes have often been implemented as part of a broader health promotion strategy, but in many low- and middle-income countries they also emerged as easy ways to raise revenues. The support of health professionals and civil society has been critical to ensure the appropriate implementation of taxes and to counteract undue pressure from the food and beverage industry.

The introduction of diet-related taxes will have to be coordinated and sequenced with other tax reforms such as VAT on goods and services. The Gulf Cooperation Council countries first introduced the VAT and then successfully added diet-related taxes. In Kerala the sequencing was the other way around, and the fat tax ended in 2017. Chile's tax was part of a tax reform package; it was not explicitly designed as a health tax and some selected SSBs actually experienced reduced taxes (Caro et al. 2018). Mexico, in contrast, included the SSB tax as a health-related tax, but the nonessential food tax was added by the Ministry of Finance to raise revenues and it was designed very rapidly with many gaps in the definition of nonessential foods.

Impact of Diet-Related Taxes

Evidence from countries with diet-related taxes shows that taxes have an impact on the consumption of unhealthy products. Studies have mainly shown the effect of diet-related taxes on the products' price and consumption, and on the population's health status. In January 2012, France introduced a tax of €7.16 per hectoliter of non-alcoholic beverages with added sugar or sweeteners, including sodas, fruit drinks, and flavored waters. Capacci et al. (2016) examined to what extent the tax was passed on to consumers through a price increase on the taxed beverages. Findings suggest that within six months soda prices increased fully by the SSB tax amount of about 11 cents for 1.5 liter of soda. However, the tax was not fully passed on to prices for fruit drinks and flavored waters, and different price increases were applied across vendors and beverages (Berardi et al. 2016). Denmark introduced a tax as a percentage of the price of soft drinks in 1998 and 2001 (Jensen and Smed 2013; Smed et al. 2016). Bergman and Hansen (2016) analyzed a micro price data set and found that both tax increases were over-shifted on to consumers—that is, the price increase for consumers was higher than the nominal value of the tax.

A tax must be high enough to trigger a change. Studies of the expected consumption effect suggest that a sales tax of around 5 percent on soft drinks tends to be too small to affect consumption (Brownell et al. 2009; Caro et al. 2018). The WHO has recommended a diet-related tax equivalent of 20 percent of the retail price to effectively change consumption. Tax simulations from Chile indicate that an 18 percent tax on ultra-processed junk foods and beverages (those high in fats, salt, sugars) is associated with the highest reduction in intake of calories, sodium, saturated fats, and added sugar, compared with alternative policies (Caro, Ng, Taillie et al. 2017). Another study from Chile found a drop of 21.6 percent in the monthly purchased volume of higher-taxed sugary soft drinks (Nakamura et al. 2018), but an alternate study using the same data set found, for the same 3.1 percent price increase, only a comparable 3 percent reduction in purchases (Caro et al. 2018). Both studies found the same small price increase but the Nakamura one found a much larger, almost unbelievable, purchase reduction from this small price increase. In Mexico, the National Public Health Institute predicted that a 10 percent increase in the price of SSBs would reduce consumption by around 10 percent, which would translate into a 12 percent reduction in new cases of diabetes. However, the first year of the tax decreased consumption by about 6 percent; the second year, purchases decreased an additional 4 percent approximately (Colchero et al. 2016; Colchero, Rivera-Dommarco et al. 2017). Similar reductions in soda consumption have been observed in the city of Berkeley, California, in response to a soda tax introduced in November 2014 (Silver et al. 2017). Most importantly, the Mexican SSB tax was associated with a much higher decline in purchases among heavy consumers—those for whom the health impact of the tax would be potentially most effective (Ng et al. 2018).

The recently introduced SSB tax in Thailand may not be high enough (the WHO recommends 20 percent) and may thus have less effect on consumer behavior. The tax will increase the final retail price by approximately 2.00 baht (US$0.06) or 10.6 percent, which is below the WHO recommended 20 percent. As noted above, the Thai Ministry of Finance plans a phased approach to increase the SSB tax rate every two years until 2023.

Colchero et al. (2016) examined pre- and post-tax purchase trends in Mexico from January 2012 to December 2014 to compare the predicted volumes of taxed and untaxed beverages purchased in 2014 with the estimated volumes that would have been purchased without the tax. Following the introduction of a tax of 1 Mexican peso per liter on any non-alcoholic beverage with added sugar in 2014, sales of sugary beverages fell on average by 6 percent. All socioeconomic groups reduced their consumption; low-income groups reported the highest reductions: they cut their sugary drink intake by 9 percent during 2014. Purchases of untaxed beverages—mainly bottled plain water—increased and were 4 percent higher than the counterfactual (Colchero et al. 2016). Similarly, studies from Hungary report reduced consumption of unhealthy products after the excise on soft and energy drinks was introduced in 2011, and most people maintained this lower consumption level over time (WHO Regional Office for Europe 2015b).

In Kerala, the government expected that the fat tax would lead to reduced consumption of unhealthy food. However, the tax was levied only on multinational chains and branded trademark owners, which comprise less than 10 percent of the food business in Kerala. Much of the unhealthy food consumed by the population of Kerala is produced by local businesses such as bakeries, food stalls, and home-grown fast food chains, but they were exempt from the fat tax. It is not clear whether the one-year fat tax has influenced food consumption and health outcomes.

Research from the European Union concludes that an excise tax based on the sugar content is the most effective way to limit consumption of SSBs (Bonnet and Réquillart 2013). Longer-term data and surveys will be needed to evaluate the impact of reduced consumption of unhealthy products on obesity and diabetes in these countries.

Diet-related taxes generate a public discourse on healthy diets. The experience with strong opposition to sin taxes from the United States shows that the campaign to pass the tax—even if unsuccessful—helps to inform consumers about unhealthy products, encourages producers to reformulate the nutrition content of products, and reduces consumption of unhealthy drinks and foods. The one-year introduction of the fat tax in Kerala has generated a public discussion in the national media about obesity and unhealthy food, although the tax has been abolished because of the introduction of the goods and services tax (GST). Following Kerala's experience, the Food Standard and Safety Authority in India set up a national committee that recommended introducing diet-related taxes on processed food with high salt and fat content. Other ideas under consideration are Chile-style front-of-package labels with negative warnings, described later in this chapter.

Because of the relatively recent experience with diet-related taxes, it is too early to identify a definitive impact on health status. Therefore, most studies report on their expected health effect. Studies from the United States suggest that a 20 percent price increase through a tax on SSBs would result in a daily reduction of 24.3 kilocalories intake per individual (Finkelstein et al. 2013). In Mexico, additional revenues from diet-related taxes were initially proposed for use in providing potable drinking water fountains in low-income schools, but this has not been implemented. Two studies have used the diet effects of the SSB tax in Mexico to project the impact over 10 and 20 years on mortality and NCDs and have found quite significant effects (Barrientos-Gutierrez et al. 2017; Sánchez-Romero et al. 2016). The first study found that the 10 percent tax on SSBs in Mexico is expected to reduce obesity by 2.5 percent by 2024 and prevent 86,000 to 134,000 new cases of diabetes by 2030; the second study, with an assumption of a larger impact, found 189,300 fewer cases of type 2 diabetes, 20,400 fewer cases of strokes and myocardial infarctions, and 18,900 fewer deaths occurring from 2013 to 2022. See box 5.1 for a summary of the impact of Mexico's diet-related taxes. Data and surveys over a longer time will be needed to confirm the taxation effect on population health.

The fiscal impact of diet-related taxes has been estimated in the United States. A tax of 1 cent per 30 milliliters of SSBs would increase the price of a 250 milliliter soda by about 8 cents and raise about US$14.9 billion in tax revenues in the first year (Brownell et al. 2009). The government of Kerala anticipated additional tax revenues per year from its fat tax of around 100 million Indian rupees (≈US$1,520,253).[3]

Challenges

One of the main lessons from countries with diet-related taxes is that industry opposition can substantially delay the SSB taxation process. In Thailand, the process took over a decade. In 2008, the Sweet Enough Network (SEN) partnered with nongovernmental organizations (NGOs) and academia, including the International Health Policy Foundation (IHPF), to develop SSB taxation ideas and held a full-day international seminar coordinated by the IHPF, with guest economist Barry Popkin and speakers from the Ministry of Finance, Mahidol University, and the Ministry of Public Health. Because of strong industry opposition arguments that taxes would not affect consumption but instead lead to job losses and negatively affect the poor, the Thai Ministry of Public Health withdrew the taxation proposal in 2011. However, by 2012, SSB-tax advocates regrouped and argued based on the successful introduction of SSB taxation in other countries, including Hungary and Mexico, and by citing increasing evidence of the effectiveness of SSB taxation on consumer behavior. In early 2016, after it had been endorsed by the National Reform Steering Assembly (NRSA), the Thai government reviewed the SSB taxation proposal again. The proposal recommended the SSB tax be limited to beverages containing sugar above 6 grams per 100 milliliters at a rate that could result in an after-tax increase of at least 20 percent on the retail price. However, the beverage and sugar industries again opposed the proposal. But this time the SSB taxation team countered the industry with research findings and media support, and with support of NGOs as well as the WHO. Ultimately, the National Reform Council (NRC) and the NRSA voted in favor of SSB taxation in 2016. In January 2017, the Thai government announced the implementation of SSB taxes in September 2017.

This was not the only Thai focus for creating healthier diets. The Thai government, led by their Food and Drug Administration and scholars from Mahidol University, met a number of times to create a front-of-package labeling system. They opted for working regionally with Singapore, Malaysia, and China in a series of meetings that ultimately led to the development in each country of positive logo choices-style front-of-package systems (Roodenburg, Popkin, and Seidell 2011). After several years of meetings, in August 2016, the voluntary Healthier Choices logo—a front-of-package labeling scheme to help consumers identify healthier food choices—was launched in Thailand.[4] The logo was developed in a collaboration between the National Food Commission, the Ministry of Public Health's Food and Drug Administration, the Health Promotion Foundation, and Mahidol University. The Healthier Choices logo is owned by the Thai Food and Drug Administration, and its use is managed by the Nutrition Promotion Foundation of Mahidol University. Industry opposition again led to this becoming voluntary rather than legally required.

In Kerala the tax was introduced swiftly. The food industry associations were not consulted about the diet-related food tax. Rather, they learned about the fat tax when the budget was announced. Still, most industry associations supported the tax as a positive step toward controlling overweight/obesity. It could also be that industry representatives may have anticipated that the fat tax would be short-lived, since the national government was preparing for the GST nationwide, which would exempt obesogenic products from taxation.

Some governments—including those of Demark, Finland, and Kerala—had to abolish their diet-related taxes for different reasons, which provide useful lessons for future consideration:

- **Denmark** introduced an excise tax of €2.15 per kilogram of saturated fat, plus an additional 25 percent ad valorem tax. Although the tax was efficient in reducing the intake of saturated fat, opponents of the tax—mainly the food industry—successfully initiated European Union (EU) jurisdictional action against it. The tax was abolished on the grounds of design weaknesses, insufficient support from public health groups, and lack of evidence that it would improve health outcomes.
- **Finland** abolished the tax on sweets in 2015 in response to pressure from the food industry, which argued that a tax on specific products is unfairly discriminatory against specific manufacturers and therefore distorting competition.
- **Kerala** abolished its fat tax after one year, in 2017, when the national government of India introduced the GST. However, the GST does not tax unhealthy food but it did place an additional sin tax on carbonated beverages of 28 percent and on processed packaged foods of an additional 12 percent GST. Unofficially no price increases have been seen in SSBs after the national government tax reforms were instituted.

These challenges highlight the need for a well-planned public awareness campaign, involving a broad coalition of health and community leaders, that can help inform the public about the potential harm caused by the taxed unhealthy products and overcome opposition to diet-related taxes. Diet-related taxes should be implemented as part of a broader health promotion strategy with the support of health professionals and civil society to ensure appropriate implementation and counteract undue pressure from the food and beverage industry. This strategy can include warning labels on taxed products to inform the public about health impacts as well as limit the marketing of taxed products to children. In addition, evidence of the effects of taxes on food purchases, consumption, population health, and revenues will help inform policy adjustments and the launch of diet-related taxes in other countries.

Lessons from Countries with Diet-Related Taxes

Countries with diet-related taxes provide important lessons for other countries that plan similar fiscal policies (Jou and Techakehakij 2012):

- First, taxes on SSBs and unhealthy foods should be developed and implemented in coordination with VAT reforms and tobacco taxes when possible. The revenue collection authority unit at the ministry of finance would be responsible for implementing diet-related taxes, and the same requirements would apply for the administration of all taxes. A realistic timeline for designing and implementing a tax will be essential to manage the process and should be aligned with ongoing tax reforms.
- The introduction of a diet-related tax would have to be sequenced appropriately to prevent overloading the tax system. Governments may consider identifying a steering committee to supervise and guide the implementation process or task the VAT steering committee with supervising the process. Legislation and regulations would have to be passed to implement a diet-related tax, and this legislation should be aligned with legislation on VAT and on tobacco taxes.
- Governments would need to consider defining the major policy issues to be addressed with diet-related taxes to develop a strategy that will serve as the basis for public dialogue. The policy issues include whether the tax will be a specific excise tax based on product volume such as liter or kilogram or nutrient content, or an ad valorem tax. Policy decisions would have to be made on the criteria to be used in nutrition profiling to decide which beverages and foods would be taxed and whether the tax should be levied on the consumer or on the producer, as is the case in the United Kingdom. The WHO nutrient profiling model can serve to identify the foods and beverages to be taxed, or a similar system could be adapted as various WHO regional offices have done (PAHO 2016). Chile created its nutrient profiling model earlier; this is highly impactful and has been adapted by Israel, Peru, and Uruguay (Colchero et al. 2016; Colchero, Rivera-Dommarco et al. 2017; Corvalán et al. 2013, 2018). This model is based on grams and milliliters of food (versus the PAHO use of milligrams of salt per 1,000 kilocalories), limited its warning labels

to four components to allow an adequate size for each logo, and did not use the labels for controversial issues (for example, diet sweeteners and total fat content) as some other profile systems have done. This approach allowed Chile and Israel to withstand many legal challenges from the industry and the World Trade Organization.

- International experience suggests that a diet-related tax should be defined as a specific excise tax based on volume and levied on either the producer or the wholesaler. As in Finland, France, Hungary, and Mexico, for example, governments may decide to charge a specific tax amount per liter of beverage with added sugar on all such beverages or per kilogram of energy-dense foods (such as candies, pastries, ice cream, chocolate, pudding, peanut butter, vegetable and palm oil products, and so on). Alternatively, the government could levy the tax per gram of sugar and fat in drinks and foods, as has been done in South Africa, leading to higher taxes on products high in sugar or fat content. Or the government can reinforce other policies and use a nutrient profiling system such as that of Chile, which identifies the most unhealthy, ultra-processed foods for taxation.

- A diet-related tax should be implemented as part of a broader strategy for healthy diets. To examine possible market reactions from the industry, a market analysis of the beverage and food industry would shed light on how they will likely react to a possible diet-related tax. Such an analysis might help gain the public support of health professionals for a tax and counteract undue pressure from the industry. In addition, a public information and education campaign involving health professionals and civil society could help inform the public about the negative health effect of sugary drinks and energy-dense foods and help prevent opposition to the tax. A public awareness campaign could also encourage healthy behavior through healthier food consumption and physical activities, particularly for children and adolescents. Food regulations through front-of-package nutrition labels would inform consumers about the nutrient content of food. As in Chile, governments could consider passing a law on food labeling that requires food labels similar to a traffic stop sign to identify products high in sugars, trans-fats, sodium, and calories (Corvalán et al. 2018). Governments would need to set up a monitoring and evaluation framework to examine the effect of taxation on purchase, consumption, revenues, and population health. Similarly, as in Mexico, population surveys could be conducted before and after the launch of the tax to evaluate possible consumption changes following the price increase. To estimate changes in consumption levels, information would have to be collected across different population groups on the consumption frequency and amount of the taxed goods and substitution goods.

- Finally, countries may want to consider developing and implementing diet-related taxes in coordination with neighboring countries. A regional approach to taxation would reduce cross-border purchases and prevent resulting tax evasion.

There are major gaps in the current sets of fiscal policies. Few countries have used the revenue for health purposes. None have considered tying the taxes to subsidies for healthier legumes, vegetables and fruits, and other healthful, less obesogenic foods. None have gone further and created targeted subsidies for healthier foods or to use subsidies to ensure increased purchases of foods such as legumes and vegetables, albeit the challenges of earmarking sin taxes for public programs brings even more challenges.

Country Experience with Other Diet-Related Programs and Policies

While fiscal policies linked mainly to SSB taxes have dominated in the response to overweight/obesity, many other regulatory options are being used by countries to achieve improved diet quality and prevent overweight/obesity. One of the newer initiatives, which was led by innovative policies in Chile, is to create a nutrient profiling model that can be linked not only to fiscal policies but also to food marketing, front-of-package food warning labels, school food bans on regulated food, and marketing controls (Corvalán et al. 2013; Corvalán et al. 2018). A series of evaluations and historical descriptions of the first 18 months of the Chilean experience will be published in the near future, possibly in 2020; it will show remarkably large impacts (Correa et al. 2019). This Chilean approach, as well as a more recently adopted recommendation by the Pan-American Health Organization (PAHO), focuses on unhealthy ultra-processed foods and beverages and attempts to shift eating norms away from these foods (PAHO 2016). Doing so may well shift food norms away from the least healthful components of ultra-processed packaged foods and beverages, but it will not necessarily push consumers to pick the least obesogenic diet. Israel plans to combine a negative warning label designed to mirror Chile's label with a positive logo on the healthiest foods and beverages such as whole grain breads, water, unsweetened dairy products, legumes, and produce (Endevelt et al. 2017). Important experimentation is expected over the next decade in an attempt to learn best practices.

Policies in this area are really in their infancy and to date no country—be it a low- or middle-income country or a high-income country—has reduced overweight/obesity, so the programs and policies that are initiated need rigorous evaluations to allow us to ultimately understand which combination of policies can create the desired food norms and ultimately create a truly healthy diet that adequately reduces the risks of being overweight/obese.

Front-of-Package Labeling

At this time a small number of countries have national regulations requiring front-of-package label profiling. A much larger number of countries across the globe have voluntary systems, as shown in map 5.5. The few countries with statutory programs are Thailand, with a positive healthier choices label (Roodenburg, Popkin, and Seidell 2011); and Chile, Israel, Peru, and Uruguay (and soon Canada), with negative warning labels (Corvalán et al. 2019). Four to six other countries are moving to utilize negative warning labels. India has already had hearings on such a negative warning label system and now is in the final phases of considering it. Israel will use both negative and positive labels in an effort to address the large proportion of foods that are not deemed very unhealthy but might not be as good for preventing overweight/obesity (for example, identifying whole grain bread versus refined carbohydrate-based breads).

There are approximately 20 to 25 other countries with some sort of voluntary front-of-package label, which vary from those promoting healthy food choices (Choices International and Scandinavian Keyhole) to traffic light systems with red, yellow, and green signals for various nutrients and those providing grading systems, such as the French Nutri-Score approach (Frølich, Åman, and Tetens 2013; Julia and Hercberg 2017; Roodenburg, Popkin, and Seidell 2011).[5]

Published evaluations to date are rare. Only the Chilean approach is being thoroughly evaluated, but this multipronged approach in Chile will not tell us whether a policy focused only on front-of-package warning labels will be effective. An evaluation of the front-of-package law is underway in Peru; this may provide further information. Maps 5.5 and 5.6 give a sense of the array of front-of-package labeling options that exist but, aside from Chile, none have been shown to impact purchasing behavior systematically (Crockett et al. 2018).

The countries with mandatory interpretive labels are much fewer than those with voluntary ones, as shown in map 5.6. Of these, the negative warning label is the one that several regional WHO groups (such as PAHO and the WHO regional offices in Latin America and Europe) are promoting.

Nutrient Profiling Models

Behind all of the front-of-package labeling approaches is some type of nutrient profiling system (Rayner, Scarborough, and Kaur 2013). Many of

Map 5.5 Countries with Mandatory or Voluntary Front-of-Package Labels

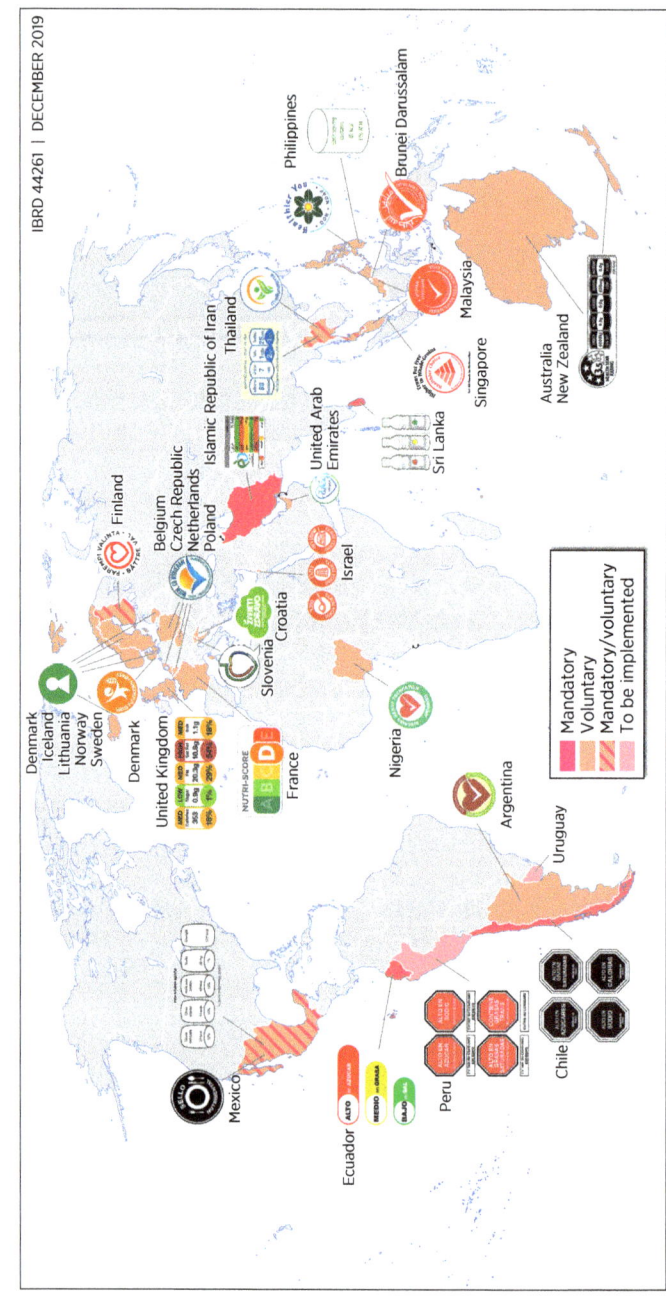

IBRD 44261 | DECEMBER 2019

Source: Global Food Research Program, University of North Carolina, 2019, http://globalfoodresearchprogram.web.unc.edu/multi-country
-initiative/resources/.

Note: The map was created based on the dataset available as of March 2019.

Map 5.6 Countries with Mandatory Front-of-Package Labels

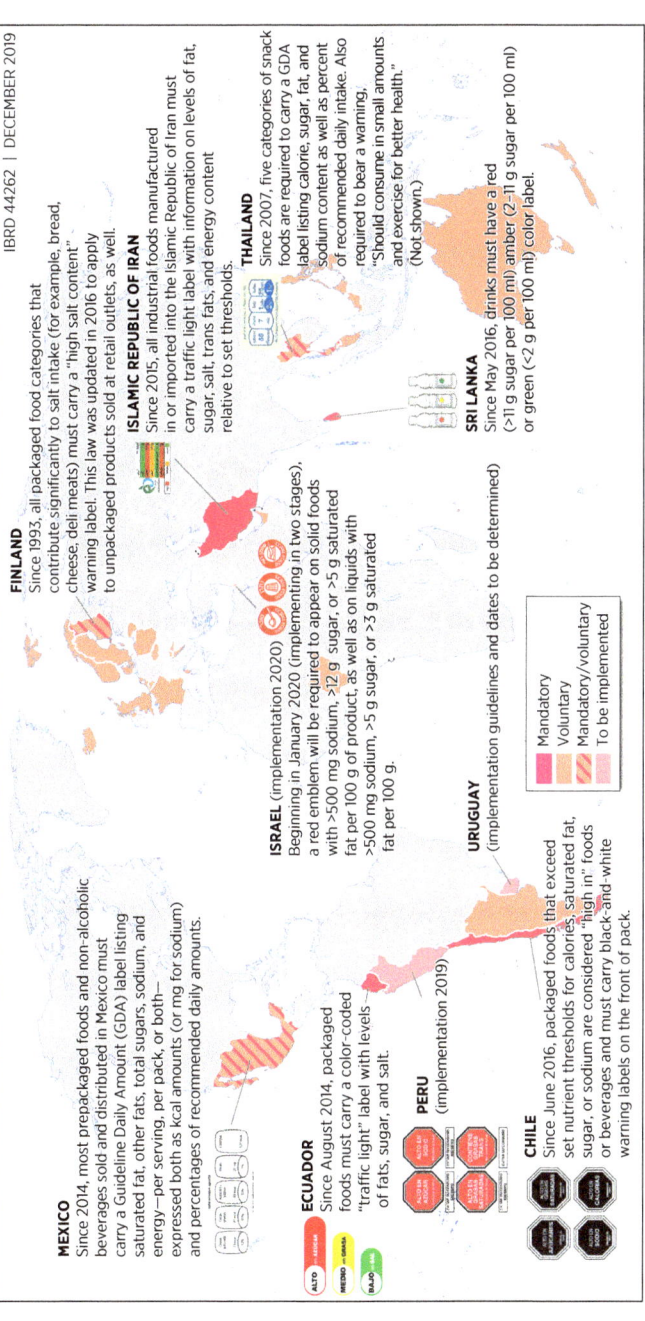

IBRD 44262 | DECEMBER 2019

MEXICO
Since 2014, most prepackaged foods and non-alcoholic beverages sold and distributed in Mexico must carry a Guideline Daily Amount (GDA) label listing saturated fat, other fats, total sugars, sodium, and energy—per serving, per pack, or both— expressed both as kcal amounts (or mg for sodium) and percentages of recommended daily amounts.

ECUADOR
Since August 2014, packaged foods must carry a color-coded "traffic light" label with levels of fats, sugar, and salt.

PERU
(implementation 2019)

CHILE
Since June 2016, packaged foods that exceed set nutrient thresholds for calories, saturated fat, sugar, or sodium are considered "high in" foods or beverages and must carry black-and-white warning labels on the front of pack.

URUGUAY
(implementation guidelines and dates to be determined)

ISRAEL (implementation 2020)
Beginning in January 2020 (implementing in two stages), a red emblem will be required to appear on solid foods with >500 mg sodium, >12 g sugar, or >5 g saturated fat per 100 g of product, as well as on liquids with >500 mg sodium, >5 g sugar, or >3 g saturated fat per 100 g.

FINLAND
Since 1993, all packaged food categories that contribute significantly to salt intake (for example, bread, cheese, deli meats) must carry a "high salt content" warning label. This law was updated in 2016 to apply to unpackaged products sold at retail outlets, as well.

ISLAMIC REPUBLIC OF IRAN
Since 2015, all industrial foods manufactured in or imported into the Islamic Republic of Iran must carry a traffic light label with information on levels of fat, sugar, salt, trans fats, and energy content relative to set thresholds.

THAILAND
Since 2007, five categories of snack foods are required to carry a GDA label listing calorie, sugar, fat, and sodium content as well as percent of recommended daily intake. Also required to bear a warning. "Should consume in small amounts and exercise for better health." (Not shown.)

SRI LANKA
Since May 2016, drinks must have a red (>11 g sugar per 100 ml) amber (2–11 g sugar per 100 ml) or green (<2 g per 100 ml) color label.

Mandatory
Voluntary
Mandatory/voluntary
To be implemented

Source: Global Food Research Program, University of North Carolina, 2019, http://globalfoodresearchprogram.web.unc.edu/multi-country-initiative/resources/.

Note: The map was created based on the dataset available as of March 2019. g = grams; GDA = Guideline Daily Amount; mg = milligrams; ml = milliliter.

the early systems were focused on creating nutrition profiles for foods that would be banned in child-focused marketing regulations. Several regional WHO offices have created their own nutrient profiling models, including WHO Europe (WHO Regional Office for Europe 2015a), PAHO (PAHO 2016), and other regional WHO offices. The Chilean government created their approach earlier (Corvalán et al. 2013; Corvalán et al. 2018) and is the only nutrient profiling approach adoped as law in other countries (for example, Israel, Peru, Uruguay). In each case, these models focus on removing nonessential or unhealthy ultra-processed foods and beverages. Many other models have been prepared based on an array of criteria, but in general they focus around one of three themes: identifying ultra-processed foods and beverages, identifying very healthy foods and beverages, and some type of grading system overall or for various nutrient components. Another useful guide for implementing a front-of-package label in a country comes from a World Cancer Research Fund document (WCRFI 2019).

The Chilean case is highly cited and used as it utilizes its nutrient profiling model not only to create a negative warning label on packaged foods but also to ban foods and beverages with the warning label from schools and to use it for a series of marketing laws. This experience has led to three countries that used the exact Chilean approach and cutoffs and a number of others that are considering front-of-package labeling laws similar to Chile's (for example, Brazil, Colombia, and Mexico).

It is increasingly felt by all involved in the areas of promoting healthier eating that such systems are essential for the design of front-of-package labeling, marketing controls, school food services and vendors selling in schools or around schools, and taxation on unhealthy foods. However, aside from Chile—where a half dozen publications to come out possibly in 2020 will identify many aspects of the impact of the Chilean approach— little will be known about the actual impact of such systems on food purchasing and overall diets. To date these comprehensive nutrient profiling models have not been utilized for fiscal policies, but at least one country is considering this.

School Food Services and Food Available at and around Schools

A large number of countries have begun to consider or already have policies banning unhealthier foods and beverages and promoting healthier eating patterns. One of the more innovative is the Brazilian approach, which puts a premium on both promoting the use of fresh foods and on small farmer employment. The Brazilian approach (Coitinho, Monteiro, and Popkin 2002), which has become a model emulated by some other countries in both Sub-Saharan Africa and Latin America, requires

30 percent of all food to be purchased from local small farmers and another 40 percent to come from real foods. No evaluations have been performed of either the employment impact or the nutritional impact of this program on food consumed at school or overall for children involved in these programs.

One key thrust in many countries is removing SSBs from schools and promoting only healthy foods and beverages to be sold or provided in school-based programs. Another relates to vendors either coming into the schools or selling near the schools. Again, a major gap is in evaluation of such efforts, although several evaluations have been initiated in new programs at the Caribbean Institute for Health Research, University of the West Indies.

Marketing Controls: Child Oriented and Overall

Only a few countries have instituted mandatory regulatory bans on marketing oriented toward children. Many are focused on child-oriented television in a selected time period or other very limited ways (the Republic of Korea, Mexico, Thailand, and Uruguay). The most comprehensive ban occurred in Chile, where the ban does the following:

- Applies to all foods and beverages
- Uses uniform nutrition criteria across categories
- Restricts all characters on packages for foods deemed unhealthy
- Adds warning logos to packaged foods high in sugar, saturated fat, sodium, or calories marketed to other audiences
- Bans advertising of unhealthy foods when 20 percent or more of the audience is younger than 14 years of age (and, starting June 2018, instituted a regulated foods marketing ban from 6am to 10pm)

This law has shifted marketing away from children's programs toward other programs. The overall exposure of children to media, which will be published in 2019 (see Carpentier et al. 2018), has been reduced somewhat, as have the child-oriented food and beverage advertisements, but the non–child-oriented advertisements have increased. The Chilean law was modified in June 2018, and now a total ban is in effect on regulated foods and beverages (those with warning labels) from 6am to 10pm; outside those hours, any marketing must include a clear warning message about the food or beverage under regulation. A future evaluation will be able to describe the added impact of this total marketing ban. One important Chilean study that is currently under review will show no impact on either employment in each food sector or overall and also no impact on real wages. Clearly the large companies that make ultra-processed foods have wide-ranging portfolios of food products to sell.

There are few countries with mandatory or statutory marketing laws. The Chilean approach is unique in first testing its impact on child-focused marketing and now in addressing total marketing of ultra-processed foods (map 5.7). An additional 30 to 45 countries have voluntary marketing codes worked out by the food and beverage industries. In all evaluations to date, these have proven ineffectual (Théodore et al. 2017).

Again, the big gaps lie in the impact of such marketing laws on knowledge, attitudes, and, ultimately, behavior. A second major question is whether it is more important to jointly institute a set of policies as Chile did or to impose separate ones, and to determine what impact a truly effective marketing law would have.

It is clear, however, that without control over the marketing of unhealthy food and beverages, which represents a large proportion of ads seen by households in all low- and middle-income countries, it is very difficult—if not impossible—to have effective nutrition education campaigns that focus on healthier eating.

Other than Chile, no country has a comprehensive marketing law at this point, but several are currently working on such a law. In contrast, dozens of countries have ineffectual voluntary industry self-regulation standards.

Map 5.7 Countries with Any Statutory Regulations on Marketing Food to Children

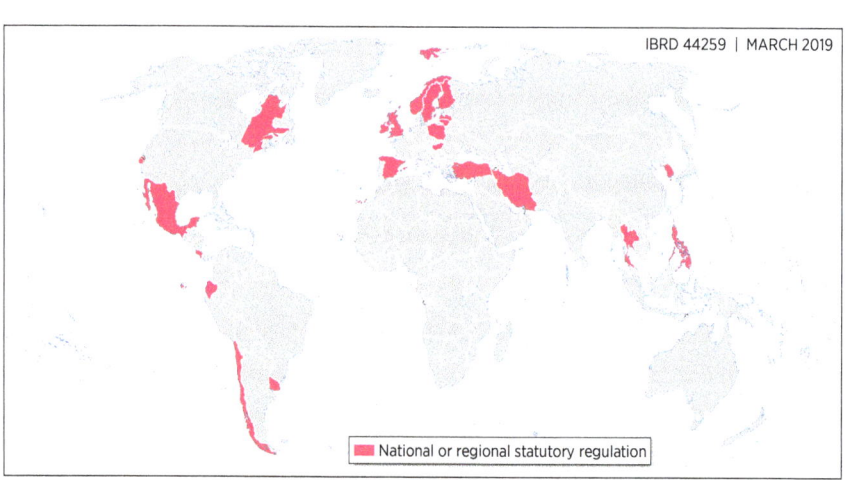

Source: Global Food Research Program, University of North Carolina, 2019, http://globalfoodresearchprogram.web.unc.edu/multi-country-initiative/resources/.

Note: The map was created based on the dataset available as of March 2019.

Retail Sector

Clearly it is the increase in the retail sector that has been responsible for opening up both households and small vendors to cheaper, quicker access to ultra-processed food (Popkin and Reardon 2018; Reardon and Berdegué 2002; Reardon et al. 2003). At the same time, improved sanitation and well-managed cold chains for handling most perishable products have resulted, and prices are often lowered—both in financial terms and in terms of time expended. There is a growing literature of small experiments in high-income countries in working with retailers to shift consumers toward healthier purchasing patterns. These experiments include shifts in the food available at checkout counters, aisle placement, provision of cold storage options to smaller stores, and in-store marketing shifts. Recently, in the United Kingdom scholars have been working with some large chains to reduce processed meat consumption, which can have both climate and health benefits. No country-level efforts have existed to date and these efforts are all very small scale. But this is a promising sector that deserves attention in low- and middle-income countries especially because retailers actually may have higher profit margins from produce and other healthier foods.

The Broader Food System

While there are many studies about the need to shift our food systems toward the promotion of healthier foods and beverages, and although the Consultative Group on International Agricultural Research (CGIAR) investment in legume and produce has increased, this sector has done relatively little to truly invest in studies on the array of credit, price, subsidy, and other policies that might be used to incentivize the entire food chain toward shifts in relative costs of healthier foods and beverages. The World Bank, the Food and Agriculture Organization of the United Nations (FAO), and many others speak about the food system and the need to promote healthier options at cheaper prices, but there are few actual impact evaluations or even process studies to show for this and no set of programs to promote globally. The World Bank's Agriculture Global Practice has expended considerable time in considering options for improving the food system (Htenas, Tanimichi-Hoberg, and Brown 2017; Townsend et al. 2016), where growing evidence shows that the entire food chain is increasingly being controlled directly by agribusinesses, food manufacturers, large retailers, and the food service sector (Popkin and Reardon 2018; Reardon, Timmer, and Minten 2012; Reardon et al. 2015).

Cross-Cutting Multisectoral Healthy Eating–Related Initiatives

In 2007 the United Kingdom produced a Foresight Report on overweight/obesity that began with a terribly complex model of all the causes of overweight/obesity. Out of this report, the government initiated across most sectors focused activities all related to promoting long-term changes in both diet and physical activity (Foresight 2007; McPherson, Marsh, and Brown 2007). Programs and policies were initiated in dozens of areas. However, a shift in governments and the cutting of funding for most of the program occurred before this effort could truly take off. This is a remarkable example, however, of how systems analysis, when linked to actual funding and program initiation in dozens of sectors, can focus on overweight/obesity prevention.

Physical Activity, Building Design, and Transportation-Related Policies

The major global push on physical activity has been to find ways to reduce sedentary behavior and increase movement and activity through urban planning, the design of the built environment, and the provision/promotion of public transport and active mobility options (box 5.2). These can range from land-use and transportation policies to integrated regional and local land-use policies and building and street design. But it is very clear we cannot remove many of the technologies that have significantly reduced activity in the economic and home sectors and in transportation. There is a much better-established literature on how various aspects of design and construction in the physical activity domain can impact movement.

While there are several reviews and broader documents on city design and physical activity (Reis et al. 2016; Sallis, Bull et al. 2016; Sallis, Cerin et al. 2016; WHO 2018), few large-scale evaluations in low- and middle-income countries show major effects on activity. Rather the literature focuses on studies of cities and areas in cities from high-income countries to document potentially important low- and middle-income country interventions. The four most important options that have the potential to be impactful are listed below. Clearly transportation and urban design as well as the education sectors are fertile areas for major impacts.

- Integrating regional and local land-use and transportation interventions can address increasing urban density, design, destination accessibility, distance to public transport, and desirability of movement in neighborhoods.

Links between Active Transport and Overweight/Obesity

Walking and bicycling, also known as active transport or nonmotorized transport, are very important modes for people to access jobs, schools, and services, especially in the cities of the developing world. Active transport has also been suggested as an option to promote physical activity and to fight both sedentarism and overweight/obesity levels, although there is very limited research to date to establish a causal link. A cross-sectional study by Evi Dons and collaborators (Dons et al. 2018) used data from seven European cities and found statistical evidence to suggest that car users have a higher body mass index (BMI) than bicycle users.

One of the fundamental reasons that active transport has been promoted as an option to reduce overweight/obesity is the low cost of the interventions (such as sidewalks and bikeways) and the possibility of targeting large user populations. In a scoping review presented by Brown et al. (2017), the authors mention that active transport can have very small impacts on BMI, but they also clarify that "active transport interventions that are low cost and targeted to those most amenable to modal switch are the most likely to be effective and cost-effective from an obesity prevention perspective." Promoting active transport in cities may therefore be a cost-effective way of controlling BMI. Since the evidence seems to point toward relatively small effects on body weight, the effectiveness of the measures will greatly depend on the size of the population being served by the interventions.

It is important to mention that promoting active modes of transport has a plethora of co-benefits that help cities achieve other health and environmental objectives beyond overweight/obesity levels. The health benefits of physical activity go beyond weight loss, with conclusive literature showing the benefits of active transport associated with mental health (Avila-Palencia et al. 2018; Mueller et al. 2015) and significant levels of reduction in all-cause mortality (Mueller et al. 2018). When an increase in bicycling and walking is promoted as modal shift from personal motorized transport, these changes also imply reductions in both greenhouse gas and local pollutant emissions (Xia et al. 2013). Despite some evidence highlighting the negative effects that higher exposures and inhaled doses of air pollutants can have on active travelers, the most recent

continued next page

Box 5.2 *(continued)*

evidence suggests that health benefits outweigh the possible negative outcomes (Tainio et al. 2016).

Promoting active transport in a safe and appropriate built environment may therefore help cities not only control the rise of overweight/obesity levels but may do so in a cost-effective way with additional co-benefits that address several Sustainable Development Goals. Few other interventions in cities can have such strong impacts across multiple development agendas.

Some of the major experiments and larger-scale studies have come from high-income countries (for example, Perth's Residential Environment work to create walkable areas and then add other facets of urban design to increase physical activity; see Giles-Corti et al. 2013; Knuiman et al. 2014). Few have been rigorously evaluated, but some lessons can be learned from these efforts.

- Promoting walking, cycling, and the use of public transport over personal motor vehicles such as cars and motorcycles is an important area of intervention with a great deal of potential. An array of cities—including many higher-income ones such as London and Stockholm—have done this; other lower-income cities such as Bogotá have also attempted this. However, none have been evaluated for impact.
- Building design that increases stair climbing by making stairs more attractive and central and escalators and elevators less attractive is another area with potential.
- Involving schools and other government facilities in these efforts can have decisive results. Schools, in particular, which have discounted the important value of activity on learning and cognitive ability as well as on health, need to rethink their curricula and experiment with wide ranges of ways to increase movement as well as provide skills in activities that can last a lifetime. In the past 20 years across the globe there has been a marked reduction in physical activity in schools as well as in facilities and equipment for physical activity, as the push to enhance learning has led to a short-sighted focus on cutting out physical activity, particularly vigorous activities.

It is important to note that in the area of physical activity improvements and overweight/obesity prevention there is a need for evaluation of large-scale urban or national programs to document their impacts on population-level activity patterns, which can in turn be linked to overweight/obesity. No evaluations equivalent to the Chilean or Mexican rigorous evaluations of their food-related fiscal and regulatory policies exist as yet in the physical activity domain.

Lessons for Overweight/Obesity Prevention Strategies from Nine Country Case Studies

The nine country case studies included for this review were developed as background papers for these analyses. They present different strategies and processes that have been implemented by governments to prevent and manage obesity among children and adults. Table 5.3 presents an overview. Most countries have some national strategy or plan to manage NCDs or overweight/obesity. School-based prevention programs are common, as childhood overweight/obesity is a growing concern globally and a predictor for overweight/obesity in adulthood.

National strategies or programs. Several governments have mandated expert groups to develop national strategies to curb overweight/obesity. Some countries, albeit not all, include overweight/obesity management as part of their broader NCD strategies. Only one country (Brazil) has focused on access to healthy, nonprocessed foods, and two of the nine (Poland and Thailand) include a focus on playgrounds for promoting physical activity.

- The Mexican government in 2010 adopted the National Agreement for Healthy Nutrition: Strategy against Overweight and Obesity (ANSA). The food and beverage industry, academia, and NGOs are all co-signatories of ANSA together with the government. ANSA established three pillars of action: (1) public health, including epidemiological surveillance, health promotion, and prevention actions; (2) medical attention, comprising quality and effective access to primary health care services; and (3) regulatory and fiscal policies in areas such as labeling, regulation of marketing strategies, and fiscal instruments to promote healthier lifestyles. The Mexican ANSA strategy includes recommendations for physical activity, safe drinking water, moderate consumption of sugars and fats in drinks, daily intake of fiber, food labeling to inform decision-making, exclusive breastfeeding, appropriate portion sizes, as well as reduced intakes of saturated fats, sodium, and added caloric sweeteners. In Mexico, the development of the national ANSA strategy has helped generate a national dialogue on overweight/obesity and put the topic on the government's agenda.

Table 5.3 Overview of Strategies and Processes to Prevent and Manage Overweight/Obesity

Strategy/Policy	Mexico	Brazil	Chile	Kerala (India)	Poland	Thailand	South Africa	Sri Lanka	Turkey
National strategy/program	X	X	Food law	NCD strategy	NCD strategy	X	X	NCD strategy	X
Initiatives for government entities	X	X				X		X	X
School-based prevention	X	X	X		X	X		X	X
Regulations on marketing and advertisement of unhealthy food and beverages	X	X	X			X			
Mass media to inform about healthy diet	X		X		X	X	X		
Food labeling	X	X	X		X	X	X	X	
Nutritional education in primary school curriculum	X	X	X						
Access to healthy, nonprocessed food markets		X							
Physical activity (playgrounds)					X	X			
School health survey screening for overweight	X	X	X		X	X			X

Note: NCD = non-communicable disease.

- Brazil takes a multisectoral approach to improve nutritional outcomes through the Intersectoral Strategy to Prevent and Control Obesity, the National Pact for Healthy Eating, and policies to ensure access to healthy food.
- Chile has perhaps the most aggressive multisectoral program to address overweight/obesity, as highlighted in the sections above.
- Kerala addresses overweight/obesity as part of its National Program for Prevention and Control of Cancer, Diabetes, Cardiovascular Diseases and Stroke (NPCDCS), which focuses on early diagnosis, treatment, and behavior change in family health centers.
- Poland introduced in 2006 the first National Program for the Prevention of Overweight and Obesity and Chronic Non-Communicable Diseases through Improved Nutrition and Physical Activity 2007–2011. In 2012, the program was extended as the National Program for the Prevention of Non-Communicable Diseases 2012–2014. Both programs highlight the role for central and local governments in health policies and prevention of NCDs.
- The Thailand Healthy Lifestyle Strategic Plan promotes healthy food consumption and physical activity.
- South Africa has the National Strategy for the Prevention and Control of Obesity (2015–2020).
- Sri Lanka developed and adopted the Multisectoral Action Plan for the Prevention and Control of Non-Communicable Diseases 2016–2020, which aims to reduce the preventable and avoidable burden of morbidity, mortality, and disability due to NCDs.
- Turkey developed the Healthy Nutrition and Active Life (HNAL) Program in 2010 to control overweight/obesity. The program aims to (1) improve equitable access to basic healthy foods for a balanced and healthy diet; (2) allocate resources to fight overweight/obesity in all sectors and to include fighting overweight/obesity in sector plans; (3) conduct an analysis of the overweight/obesity situation in Turkey for different population groups; and (4) establish a monitoring and evaluation system to regularly track overweight/obesity progression.

Countries such as Chile that have put in place multipronged strategies are starting to show results (figure 5.1).

Initiatives. In line with national strategies and agreements, governments have established various initiatives for government agencies to regulate unhealthy dietary intake. Initiatives include policies and actions to be implemented across different government entities. For example, the Fatless Belly Thais policy in Thailand includes various initiatives for different government agencies to implement, and Sri Lanka has set up the Nutrition Coordination Division within its Ministry of Health. Mexico's Health

Figure 5.1   Chile's Multipronged Obesity Prevention Program

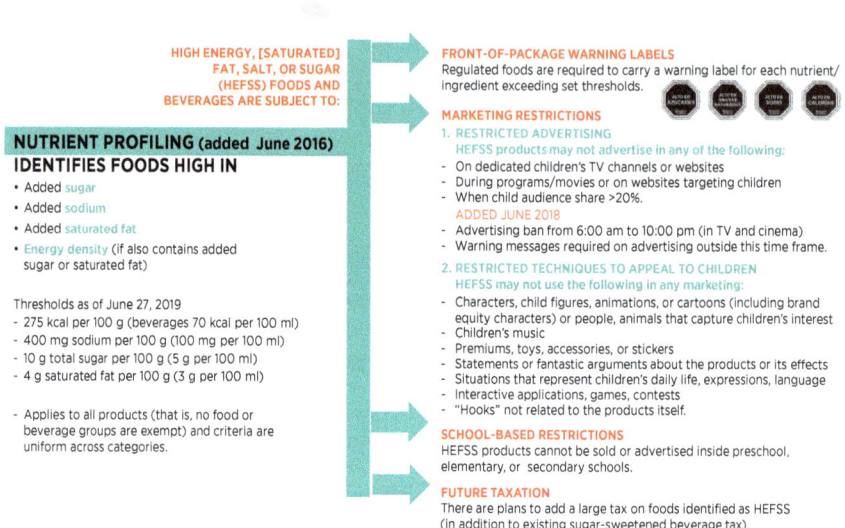

Source: Institute of Nutrition and Food Technology, University of Chile and Global Food Research Program, University of North Carolina.

Note: g = grams; HEFSS = high energy, saturated fat, salt, or sugar; kcal = kilocalorie; mg = milligrams; ml = milliliter.

Secretariat launched a National Strategy for the Prevention and Control of Overweight, Obesity, and Diabetes signed by the president and all cabinet secretaries (Bonilla-Chacín et al. 2016). Brazil used a wide-ranging consultative process to establish several initiatives, the most far-reaching being the school feeding initiative to enhance fresh food use in school meals (Coitinho, Monteiro, and Popkin 2002). In 2011, Turkey created a Healthy Nutrition and Active Life Program.

School-based prevention programs. To manage overweight/obesity early on, governments have introduced school-based childhood overweight/obesity prevention programs that can include policies for healthy food and food service practices, restricted access to unhealthy food, physical education, student health services, and staff health and nutrition.

- In Mexico, the Ministry of Education has issued school guidelines to regulate the sale and distribution of foods and drinks in schools and promote healthy eating.
- The School Meal Program Law in Brazil requires healthy ingredients in meals and 30 percent of the school meal budget to be spent on healthy

fresh food produced by local farmers. SSBs are not allowed as part of school meals in Brazil.

- Chile's Food Law restricts the type of food that can be sold and distributed within schools.
- Poland regulates school food including the type of food sold in school cafeterias and shops.
- Thailand has a soda ban policy in schools for SSBs.
- In Sri Lanka, the School Canteen Program aims to prevent and control overweight/obesity by providing healthy food to children.
- Turkey has two school-based interventions that were initiated by the Ministry of Health: restrictions on the type of food and beverages sold in school canteens and a Physical Fitness Scorecard for Health to encourage physical activity among children in secondary and high schools through personalized fitness schemes.

School-based programs have not been evaluated in these countries. However, studies from the United States find encouraging results for school-based programs that combine diet and physical activity (Hung et al. 2015; Wang et al. 2015). A meta-analysis of 27 programs found that school-based interventions have not been effective for improving body mass index or curbing childhood overweight/obesity; however, programs that focused on physical activity or nutrition have shown promising results (Hung et al. 2015). Another meta-analysis of 115 school-based studies from the United States came to similar conclusions, with stronger evidence when physical activity–only interventions were delivered in schools with home involvement or diet and physical activity interventions were combined and delivered in schools with both home and community components (Wang et al. 2015).

Laws and regulations on marketing and advertisement. Regulations aim to restrict food and beverage advertisements on television during family program times and in movie theaters. In Mexico, only products meeting nutritional standards can be advertised during screen time appropriate for children, including on television and in movie theaters. Brazil mandated warning messages of health risks to accompany advertisements for unhealthy foods and beverages; however, this regulation was challenged in court by the food industry and had to be abolished. Chile also initially prohibited unhealthy food advertisement directed at children under 14 years, which has been modified as a total marketing ban on regulated foods through any media form from 6:00 am to 10:00 pm daily. Unhealthy food cannot be sold or distributed in nurseries, elementary schools, or high schools and it is forbidden to give it for free to children. In South Africa, the Advertising Standards Authority (ASA) regulates the advertisement and marketing of unhealthy food and beverages.

The ASA prohibits misleading food marketing and advertisement tactics via any form of media, including enticing children with toys and using celebrities and cartoon characters to advertise unhealthy food products to children. Some lessons from the marketing of infant formula may also apply here.

Food labeling. Regulations on food labels require that food products provide information about their content. In Chile, the Food Law requires front-of-package labeling with nutrition information clearly identifying products high in sugar, saturated fat, sodium, or calories (Corvalán et al. 2019). Foods high in sugar have more than 10 grams of sugar per 100 grams of food; foods high in saturated fat have more than 4 grams of saturated fat per 100 grams of food; those high in sodium have more than 400 milligrams of sodium per 100 grams of food, and foods are considered high in calories if 100 grams of food exceeds 275 kilocalories. For liquids, the thresholds are per 100 milliliters: 5 grams for sugar, 3 grams for saturated fat, 100 milligrams for sodium, and 70 kilocalories for energy drinks. In Sri Lanka, the food labeling and advertising regulations require that packaged food have the required food labeling. The Food Based Dietary Guidelines for Sri Lankans 2011 recommends an intake of no more than 25 grams of sugar per day per person. The Food Color Coding Regulation was enacted in 2016. Traffic light colors—green, amber (yellow), and red—are now used on the label to indicate low, medium, and high levels, respectively, of sugar. Implementation of the regulations is monitored by Public Health Inspectors and Food and Drug Inspectors. Thailand instituted a Healthy Choice–type voluntary front-of-package labeling program in 2016 patterned after the Choices International Program and the Smart Choice program used in Singapore (Foo et al. 2013; Roodenburg, Popkin, and Seidell 2011). Peru, in 2019, started a program identical to the Chilean warning label system; Israel will follow in 2020 (Endevelt et al. 2017). Both start with the Chilean second phase's more stringent lower added sodium, added saturated fat, and added sugar cutoffs.

Information through mass media. Governments and social health insurers have used mass media such as television and radio to inform the population about prevention of overweight/obesity. Mexico has added information sessions for people who visit employment centers and health care facilities. The Fatless Belly Thais policy creates public awareness about diet and physical activity through mass media and through cross-sectoral collaboration. Visual versions of dietary guidelines help ensure easy understanding across socioeconomic groups.

Nutritional education. Nutritional guidelines in school curricula have been issued by ministries of health and have become part of the curriculum in primary schools in Mexico, Brazil, and Chile. Both foods and beverages are included.

Access to healthy, nonprocessed food. Access to healthy food influences dietary behavior. Brazil has issued guidelines to improve equity in access to healthy food, particularly in low-income areas and in schools. Guidelines promote family farming, sustainable farming methods, and agriculture marketing, and they facilitate access to food markets in low-income areas.

Physical activity. The Ministry of Sports in Poland has introduced a national initiative to increase opportunities for physical activity in all communities, including the construction of playgrounds for children, soccer and basketball fields, and so on. Thailand promotes regular physical activity through national policy including public and private sector platforms to promote exercise and physical activity close to home, workplace, and community. The focus is on public parks, the mass transport system, and urban development to encourage exercise and activity.

School health surveys. Countries conduct regular national school health surveys to monitor children's health status.

- The 2008 school health survey in Mexico identified a high prevalence of overweight in children, which led to the development of the national strategy ANSA.
- The school health survey in Brazil is mandated by law and helps policy makers monitor students' nutrition status and health behavior and inform school health policies.
- The Polish Gdańsk region introduced overweight screening and intense case management for children in elementary and middle schools. Children with a BMI above the 85th percentile receive one year of case management, including four visits with health care providers (pediatrician, dietician, psychologist, and physical activity trainer) and workshops on nutrition and physical activity for children and their families.
- Turkey conducted the Childhood Obesity Initiative survey in 2013, which found an increase in childhood overweight/obesity among all age groups.

Key Interventions with Potential for Impact

Policies that restrict unhealthy foods and beverages tend to be challenged by the food and beverage industry and by stakeholders when they face difficulties finding consensus on the types of foods and beverages to be restricted. As there are no internationally recommended threshold levels for sugar intake, the process for establishing parameters for products with low, medium, or high sugar content can become challenging.

The implementation of strategies and guidelines requires budgets, implementation support, and monitoring and evaluation to ensure they achieve their objective and allow adjustments. For example, insufficient budgetary resources, poor collaboration, and inadequate monitoring and evaluation have contributed to less effective guidelines in Mexico. In Poland, the lack of human and financial resources has limited program implementation, and the school meal guidelines were too technical and restrictive and were not accurately communicated. Moreover, local food vendors were not adequately informed so they could adjust their supplies in time. As a result, children reacted by bringing their own foods and beverages to school. Guidelines were adjusted to be less restrictive on ingredients such as sugar and salt content. The soda ban policy in schools in Thailand does not ban unhealthy foods, and it does not apply to vendors near schools.

Table 5.4 provides a summary of an actionable policy agenda based on the evidence and experience of the countries discussed in this chapter. Based on our current knowledge of each item, we assess its potential impact as well as the population that can be reached by each policy.

Table 5.4 Key Interventions with Potential for Impact

Policy Intervention type	Goal	Effectiveness demonstrated	Potential impact and scope of impact on target population
Fiscal policies			
Taxes/subsidies	Reduce consumption of ultra-processed foods and beverages, primary focus to date on sugar-sweetened beverage reduction	Chile, Mexico, United Kingdom, and South Africa [papers forthcoming]; U.S. cities	• Impact depends on the size/ design of the tax • Nutrient-based taxes such as tiered taxes and taxes based on number of grams of sugar promote reformulation • Impactful in reducing consumption among high-volume consumers, with potential for prevention of overweight/obesity among children/adolescents
Regulatory policies on marketing and advertising			
Front-of-package warning labels	Reduce consumption of ultra-processed foods and beverages; change eating norms	Chile [unpublished series of papers forthcoming]	• Very impactful when combined with other linked policies • Universal targeting

continued next page

Table 5.4 (*continued*)

Policy		Effectiveness	Potential impact and scope of
Intervention type	**Goal**	**demonstrated**	**impact on target population**
Marketing controls on foods for children	Reduce consumption of ultra-processed foods and beverages; change eating norms	Chile, many others	• Potential for impact when linked to other policies • Can reduce child exposure; total family exposure does not change
Regulations on total marketing and sales of unhealthy foods	Reduce consumption of ultra-processed foods and beverages; change eating norms	Chile	• Potential for changing norms • Reaches all children; more impactful on younger children
Retailer interventions	Reduce consumption of ultra-processed foods and beverages	United States, United Kingdom	• Potential for high impact • Potential for important food purchase changes
Agriculture/food systems approaches			
Agriculture research	Incentivize research on underserved foods (legumes, fruits, vegetables)	CGIAR	• Potential for high impact • Potential to shift relative prices
	Ensure agriculture research has a nutrition focus, not just a yield focus	CGIAR, country programs	• Potential high in general; only initial stages of efforts globally • Potential huge for shifting relative food prices
Agriculture subsidies	Eliminate subsidies for unhealthy ingredients (for example, sugar, corn, palm oil)	Yet to be implemented	• Potential impact unclear for shifting relative prices; but could provide fiscal benefits for countries
Food processing	Build awareness of unhealthy ingredients used in food processing	Yet to be implemented	• Potential impact unclear

continued next page

Table 5.4 *(continued)*

Policy Intervention type	Goal	Effectiveness demonstrated	Potential impact and scope of impact on target population
Formal food service sector	Reduce consumption of ultra-processed foods and beverages	None	• Potentially impactful • As income increases, the proportion of meals eaten outside the home increases rapidly, so the potential impact rises • Dependent on laws impacting pricing policies, labeling, sizing
Informal food service sector	Reduce consumption of ultra-processed foods and beverages	Singapore	• Great potential but requires experimentation (existing experience shows limited impact as focus is on sanitation, healthy oils; no pricing/portion controls used)
Education sector approaches			
School food service quality and school premises sales regulations	Reduce consumption of ultra-processed foods and beverages; change eating norms for children	CGIAR, country programs	• Potential high; only initial stages of efforts globally • Potential huge for shifting relative food prices
Active transport and building/city design			
Mass transit system	Increase movement, energy expenditure	None	• Minimal potential for impact on overweight/obesity but important for health and climate • Mostly affects low- and middle-income populations
City design: parks, cycling lanes	Increase movement, energy expenditure	Colombia, Netherlands, United Kingdom	• Potential for impact among users
Building design to enhance walking	Increase movement, energy expenditure	Europe, United States, Australia	• Minimal impact on overweight/obesity but important for health • Potential for increasing physical activity

continued next page

Table 5.4   *(continued)*

Policy Intervention type	Goal	Effectiveness demonstrated	Potential impact and scope of impact on target population
Early childhood nutrition programs			
Breastfeeding promotion	Improve breastfeeding rates	Many countries	• Impact global as documented across many low-, middle-, and high-income countries
Prevention of early childhood stunting	Well-documented package of interventions across sectors	Many countries	• Relevant mostly for low-income countries and some middle-income countries

Note: CGIAR = Consultative Group on International Agricultural Research.

Applying the right combinations of policies and interventions in the right country context seems to be key to success. Furthermore, building national capacity to design, monitor, and implement these interventions, as well as documenting their experiences and impacts, is critical to continue to build the evidence base of what works under different contexts.

Notes

1. Further information about the Health Promotion Levy on Sugary Beverages in South Africa is available at http://www.sars.gov.za/ClientSegments /Customs-Excise/Excise/Pages/Health%20Promotion%20Levy%20on%20 Sugary%20Beverages.aspx.
2. Details about the Philadelphia beverage tax can be found at https://www .phila.gov/services/payments-assistance-taxes/business-taxes/philadelphia -beverage-tax/.
3. Per the exchange rate of April 19, 2018, US$1 equals 65.68 Indian rupees.
4. Details about the Choices Programme can be found at https://www .choicesprogramme.org/.
5. The French Nutri-Score is a system that gives all foods a grade from A to E based on a complex diet quality scoring system (Julia and Herchberg 2017).

References

Alvarado, M., N. Unwin, S. J. Sharp, I. Hambleton, M. M. Murphy, T. A. Samuels, M. Suhrcke, and J. Adams. 2019. "Assessing the Impact of the Barbados Sugar-Sweetened Beverage Tax on Beverage Sales: An Observational Study." *International Journal of Behavioral Nutrition and Physical Activity* 16 (1): 13.

Avila-Palencia,I., L. I. Panis, E. Dons, M. Gaupp-Berghausen, E. Raser, T. Götschi, R. Gerike, C. Brand, A. de Nazelle, J. P. Orjuela, E. Anaya-Boig, E. Stigell, S. Kahlmeier, F. Iacorossi, and M. J. Nieuwenhuijsen. 2018. "The Effects of Transport Mode Use on Self-Perceived Health, Mental Health, and Social Contact Measures: A Cross-Sectional and Longitudinal Study." *Environment International* 120 (2018): 199–206.

Azar, A. 2018. *Development and Implementation Processes of the Food Labeling and Advertising Law in Chile.* Global Delivery Initiative. Washington, DC: World Bank.

Barrientos-Gutierrez, T., R. Zepeda-Tello, E. R. Rodrigues, A. Colchero-Aragonés, R. Rojas-Martínez, E. Lazcano-Ponce, M. Hernández-Ávila, J. Rivera-Dommarco, and R. Meza. 2017. "Expected Population Weight and Diabetes Impact of the 1-Peso-Per-Litre Tax to Sugar Sweetened Beverages in Mexico." *PLOS ONE* 12 (5): e0176336.

Batis, C., J. A. Rivera, B. M. Popkin, and L. S. Taillie. 2016. "First-Year Evaluation of Mexico's Tax on Nonessential Energy-Dense Foods: An Observational Study." *PLOS Medicine* 13 (7): e1002057.

Begg, D., S. Fischer, and R. Dornbusch. 2000. *Economics* (6th ed). New York: McGraw-Hill.

Berardi, N., P. Sevestre, M. Tepaut, and A. Vigneron. 2016. "The Impact of a 'Soda Tax' on Prices: Evidence from French Micro Data." *Applied Economics* 48 (41): 3976–94.

Bergman, U., and N. Lynggård Hansen. 2016. "Are Excise Taxes on Beverages Fully Passed through to Prices? The Danish Evidence." FinanzArchiv 10.1628/fa-2019-0010.

Bonilla-Chacín, M. E., R. Iglesias, A. Suaya, C. Trezza, and C. Macías. 2016. "Learning from the Mexican Experience with Taxes on Sugar-Sweetened Beverages and Energy-Dense Foods of Low Nutritional Value: Poverty and Social Impact Analysis." Health, Nutrition and Population Discussion Paper. World Bank, Washington, DC.

Bonnet, C., and V. Réquillart. 2013. "Tax Incidence with Strategic Firms in the Soft Drink Market." *Journal of Public Economics* 106: 77–88.

Briggs, A. D. M., O. T. Mytton, A. Kehlbacher, R. Tiffin, A. Elhussein, M. Rayner, S. A. Jebb, T. Blakely, and P. Scarborough. 2017. "Health Impact Assessment of the UK Soft Drinks Industry Levy: A Comparative Risk Assessment Modelling Study." *The Lancet Public Health* 2 (1): e15–e22.

Brown, V., M. Moodie, A. M. Mantilla Herrera, J. L. Veerman, and R. Carter. 2017. "Active Transport and Obesity Prevention: A Transportation Sector Obesity Impact Scoping Review and Assessment for Melbourne, Australia." *Preventive Medicine* 96: 49–66.

Brownell, K. D., T. Farley, W. C. Willett, B. M. Popkin, F. J. Chaloupka, J. W. Thompson, and D. S. Ludwig. 2009. "The Public Health and Economic Benefits of Taxing Sugar-Sweetened Beverages." *New England Journal of Medicine* 361 (16): 1599–605.

Capacci, S., O. Allais, C. Bonnet, and M. Mazzocchi. 2016. "The Impact of the French Soda Tax on Prices and Purchases: An Ex Post Evaluation." Preliminary paper. https://www.aeaweb.org/conference/2019/preliminary/paper/Ni9ZDaQD.

Caro, J. C., C. Corvalán, M. Reyes, A. Silva, B. Popkin, and L. S. Taillie. 2018. "Chile's 2014 Sugar-Sweetened Beverage Tax and Changes in Prices and Purchases of Sugar-Sweetened Beverages: An Observational Study in an Urban Environment." *PLOS Medicine* 15 (7): e1002597.

Caro, J. C., S. W. Ng, R. Bonilla, J. Tovar, and B. M. Popkin. 2017. "Sugary Drinks Taxation, Projected Consumption and Fiscal Revenues in Colombia: Evidence from a QUAIDS Model." *PLOS One*, December 20. https://doi.org/10.1371/journal.pone.0189026.

Caro, J. C., S. W. Ng, L. S. Taillie, and B. M. Popkin. 2017. "Designing a Tax to Discourage Unhealthy Food and Beverage Purchases: The Case of Chile." *Food Policy* 71: 86–100.

Carpentier, F., T. Correa, M. Reyes, and L. Taillie. 2018. "Preschool and Adolescent Children's Changes in Exposure to Food Advertising on Television: Evaluating the Impact of Chile's Marketing Regulation of Unhealthy Foods and Beverages." Presentation at the Latin American Nutrition Society Congress (SLAN), Guadalajara, November 11–15.

Cawley, J., D. Frisvold, A. Hill, and D. Jones. 2018. "The Impact of the Philadelphia Beverage Tax on Purchases and Consumption by Adults and Children." NBER Working Paper 25052. National Bureau of Economic Research, Cambridge, MA. https://www.nber.org/papers/w25052.

Cediel, G., M. Reyes, M. L. da Costa Louzada, E. Martinez Steele, C. A. Monteiro, C. Corvalán, and R. Uauy. 2017. "Ultra-Processed Foods and Added Sugars in the Chilean Diet (2010)." *Public Health Nutrition* 21 (1): 125–33.

Chakrabarti, S., A. Kishore, and D. Roy. 2018. "Effectiveness of Food Subsidies in Raising Healthy Food Consumption: Public Distribution of Pulses In India." *American Journal of Agricultural Economics* 100 (5): 1427–49.

Coitinho, D., C. A. Monteiro, and B. M. Popkin. 2002. "What Brazil Is Doing to Promote Healthy Diets and Active Lifestyles." *Public Health Nutrition* 5 (1A): 263–67.

Colchero, M. A., B. M. Popkin, J. A. Rivera, and S. W. Ng. 2016. "Beverage Purchases from Stores in Mexico under the Excise Tax on Sugar Sweetened Beverages: Observational Study." *BMJ* 352: h6704.

Colchero, M. A., J. Rivera-Dommarco, B. M. Popkin, and S. W. Ng. 2017. "In Mexico, Evidence of Sustained Consumer Response Two Years after Implementing a Sugar-Sweetened Beverage Tax." *Health Affairs* 36 (3): 564–71.

Colchero, M. A., J. C. Salgado, M. Unar-Munguía, M. Hernández-Ávila, and J. A. Rivera-Dommarco. 2015. "Price Elasticity of the Demand for Sugar Sweetened Beverages and Soft Drinks in Mexico." *Economics and Human Biology* 19: 129–37.

Colchero, M. A., J. C. Salgado, M. Unar-Munguía, M. Molina, S. Ng, and J. A. Rivera-Dommarco. 2015. "Changes in Prices After an Excise Tax to Sweetened Sugar Beverages Was Implemented in Mexico: Evidence from Urban Areas." *PLOS ONE* 10 (12): e0144408.

Colchero, M. A., J. A. Zavala, C. Batis, T. Shamah-Levy, and J. A. Rivera-Dommarco. 2017. "Changes in Prices of Taxed Sugar-Sweetened Beverages and Nonessential Energy Dense Food in Rural and Semi-Rural Areas in Mexico." *Salud Pública de México* 59 (2): 137–46.

Correa, T., C. Fierro, M. Reyes, F. R. Dillman Carpentier, L. S. Taillie, and C. Corvalan. 2019. "Responses to the Chilean Law of Food Labeling and Advertising: Exploring Knowledge, Perceptions and Behaviors of Mothers of Young Children." *International Journal of Behavioral Nutrition and Physical Activity* 16 (1): 21.

Corvalán, C., M. Reyes, M. L. Garmendia, and R. Uauy. 2013. "Structural Responses to the Obesity and Non-Communicable Diseases Epidemic: The Chilean Law of Food Labeling and Advertising." *Obesity Reviews* 14: 79–87.

———. 2018. "Structural Responses to the Obesity and Non-Communicable Diseases Epidemic: Update on the Chilean Law of Food Labelling and Advertising." *Obesity Reviews* 20 (3): 367–74.

Crockett, R. A., S. E. King, T. M. Marteau, A. T. Prevost, G. Bignardi, N. W. Roberts, B. Stubbs, G. J. Hollands, and S. A. Jebb. 2018. "Nutritional Labelling for Healthier Food or Non-Alcoholic Drink Purchasing and Consumption." *The Cochrane Library.*

de Walque, D. 2018. "The Use of Financial Incentives to Prevent Undesirable Behaviors." Policy Research Working Paper 8424, Washington, DC, World Bank.

DiMeglio, D. P., and R. D. Mattes. 2000. "Liquid Versus Solid Carbohydrate: Effects on Food Intake and Body Weight." *International Journal of Obesity and Related Metabolic Disorders* 24 (6): 794–800.

Dons, E., D. Rojas-Rueda, E. Anaya-Boig, I. Avila-Palencia, C. Brand, T. Cole-Hunter, A. de Nazelle, U. Eriksson, M. Gaupp-Berghausen, R. Gerike, S. Kahlmeier, M. Laeremans, N. Mueller, T. Nawrot, M. J. Nieuwenhuijsen, J. P. Orjuela, F. Racioppi, E. Raser, A. Standaert, L. I. Panis, and T. Götschi. 2018. "Transport Mode Choice and Body Mass Index: Cross-Sectional and Longitudinal Evidence from a European-Wide Study." *Environment International* 119 (October): 109–16.

Du, M., A. Tugendhaft, A. Erzse, and K. J. Hofman. 2018. "Focus: Nutrition and Food Science: Sugar-Sweetened Beverage Taxes: Industry Response and Tactics." *Yale Journal of Biology and Medicine* 91 (2): 185.

Endevelt, R., I. Grotto, R. Sheffer, R. Goldsmith, M. Golan, J. Mendlovic, and M. Bar-Siman-Tov. 2017. "Policy and Practice: Regulatory Measures to Improve the Built Nutrition Environment for Prevention of Obesity and Related Morbidity in Israel." *Public Health Panorama* 3 (4): 567–75.

Falbe, J., N. Rojas, A. H. Grummon, and K. A. Madsen. 2015. "Higher Retail Prices of Sugar-Sweetened Beverages 3 Months after Implementation of an Excise Tax in Berkeley, California." *American Journal of Public Health* 105 (11): 2194–201.

Falbe, J., H. R. Thompson, C. M. Becker, N. Rojas, C. E. McCulloch, and K. A. Madsen. 2016. "Impact of the Berkeley Excise Tax on Sugar-Sweetened Beverage Consumption." *American Journal of Public Health* 106 (10): 1865–71.

Finkelstein, E. A., C. Zhen, M. Bilger, J. Nonnemaker, A. M. Farooqui, and J. E. Todd. 2013. "Implications of a Sugar-Sweetened Beverage (SSB) Tax When Substitutions to Non-Beverage Items Are Considered." *Journal of Health Economics* 32 (1): 219–39.

Fletcher, J. 2011. "Soda Taxes and Substitution Effects: Will Obesity Be Affected?" *Choices* 26 (3): 1–4.

Fletcher, J., D. Frisvold, and N. Tefft. 2013. "Substitution Patterns Can Limit the Effects of Sugar-Sweetened Beverage Taxes on Obesity." *Preventing Chronic Disease* 10.

Foo, L. L., K. Vijaya, R. A. Sloan, and A. Ling. 2013. "Obesity Prevention and Management: Singapore's Experience." *Obesity Reviews* 14: 106–13.

Foresight. 2007. *Tackling Obesities: Future Choices-Project Report.* Government Office for Science.

Frølich, W., P. Åman, and I. Tetens. 2013. "Whole Grain Foods and Health: A Scandinavian Perspective." *Food and Nutrition Research* 57 (1): 18503.

Giles-Corti, B., F. Bull, M. Knuiman, G. McCormack, K. Van Niel, A. Timperio, H. Christian, S. Foster, M. Divitini, N. Middleton, and B. Boruff. 2013. "The Influence of Urban Design on Neighbourhood Walking Following Residential Relocation: Longitudinal Results from the RESIDE Study." *Social Science and Medicine* 77 (January): 20–30.

Guerrero-López, C. M., M. Molina, and M. A. Colchero. 2017. "Employment Changes Associated with the Introduction of Taxes on Sugar-Sweetened Beverages and Nonessential Energy-Dense Food in Mexico." *Preventive Medicine* 105: S43–S49.

Hall, K. D. 2019. "Ultra-Processed Diets Cause Excess Calorie Intake and Weight Gain: A One-Month Inpatient Randomized Controlled Trial of Ad Libitum Food Intake." *Cell Metabolism* 30: 1–10.

Härkänen, T., K. Kotakorpi, P. Pietinen, J. Pirttilä, H. Reinivuo, and I. Suoniemi. 2014. "The Welfare Effects of Health-Based Food Tax Policy." *Food Policy* 49: 196–206.

Htenas, A. M., Y. Tanimichi-Hoberg, and L. Brown. 2017. *An Overview of Links between Obesity and Food Systems: Implications for the Agriculture GP Agenda.* Washington, DC: World Bank Group.

Hung, L.-S., D. K. Tidwell, M. E. Hall, M. L. Lee, C. A. Briley, and B. P. Hunt. 2015. "A Meta-Analysis of School-Based Obesity Prevention Programs Demonstrates Limited Efficacy of Decreasing Childhood Obesity." *Nutrition Research.* 35 (3): 229–40.

IMF (International Monetary Fund). 2016. "Fiscal Policy: How to Design and Enforce Tobacco Excises?" How-To Notes. Fiscal Affairs Department, International Monetary Fund, Washington, DC.

Jacobs, A., and M. Richtel. 2017a. "A Nasty, NAFTA-Related Surprise: Mexico's Soaring Obesity." *The New York Times*, December 11. https://www.nytimes.com/2017/12/11/health/obesity-mexico-nafta.html.

———. 2017b. "She Took on Colombia's Soda Industry. Then She Was Silenced." *The New York Times*, November 13. https://www.nytimes.com/2017/11/13/health/colombia-soda-tax-obesity.html.

Jensen, J. D., and S. Smed. 2013. "The Danish Tax on Saturated Fat: Short Run Effects on Consumption, Substitution Patterns and Consumer Prices of Fats." *Food Policy* 42 (October): 18–31.

Jou, J., and W. Techakehakij. 2012. "International Application of Sugar-Sweetened Beverage (SSB) Taxation in Obesity Reduction: Factors that May Influence Policy Effectiveness in Country-Specific Contexts." *Health Policy* 107 (1): 83–90.

Julia, C., and S. Hercberg. 2017. "Development of a New Front-of-Pack Nutrition Label in France: The Five-Colour Nutri-Score." *Public Health Panorama* 3(4): 712–25.

Knuiman, M. W., H. E. Christian, M. L. Divitini, S. A. Foster, F. C. Bull, H. M. Badland, and B. Giles-Corti. 2014. "A Longitudinal Analysis of the Influence of the Neighborhood Built Environment on Walking for Transportation: The RESIDE Study." *American Journal of Epidemiology* 180 (5): 453–61.

Malik, V. S., and F. B. Hu. 2015. "Fructose and Cardiometabolic Health: What the Evidence from Sugar-Sweetened Beverages Tells Us." *Journal of the American College of Cardiology* 66 (14): 1615–24.

McPherson, K., T. Marsh, and M. Brown. 2007. "Foresight Report on Obesity." *The Lancet* 370 (9601): 1755; author reply 1755.

Mourao, D., J. Bressan, W. Campbell, and R. Mattes. 2007. "Effects of Food Form on Appetite and Energy Intake in Lean and Obese Young Adults." *International Journal of Obesity* 31 (11): 1688–95.

Mueller, N., D. Rojas-Rueda, T. Cole-Hunter, A. de Nazelle, E. Dons, R. Gerike, T. Götschi, L. I. Panis, S. Kahlmeier, and M. Nieuwenhuijsen. 2015. "Health Impact Assessment of Active Transportation: A Systematic Review." *Preventive Medicine* 76 (2015): 103–14.

Mueller, N., D. Rojas-Rueda, M. Salmona, D. Martineza, A. Ambrosa, C. Brand, A. de Nazelle, E. Dons, M. Gaupp-Berghausen, R. Gerike, T. Götschi, F. Iacorossi, L. I. Panis, S. Kahlmeier, E. Raser, and M. Nieuwenhuijsen on behalf of the PASTA consortium. 2018. "Health Impact Assessment of Cycling Network Expansions in European Cities." *Preventive Medicine* 109 (2018): 62–70.

Nair, A.B., and M. K. Suresh. Forthcoming. *The "Fat Tax" in Kerala State, India: A Case Study.*

Nakamura, R., A. Mirelman, C. Cuadrado, N. Silva, J. Dunstan, and M. E. Suhrcke. 2018. "Evaluating the 2014 Sugar-Sweetened Beverage Tax in Chile: An Observational Study in Urban Areas." *PLOS Medicine.* https://doi.org/10.1371/journal.pmed.1002596.

National Treasury, R. o. S. A. 2016. *Taxation of Sugar Sweetened Beverages*, R. o. S. A. National Treasury, Economics Tax Analysis Chief Directorate Pretoria, National Department of Treasury.

Ng, S. W., J. A. Rivera, B. M. Popkin, and M. A. Colchero. 2018. "Did High Sugar-Sweetened Beverage Purchasers Respond Differently to the Excise Tax on Sugar-Sweetened Beverages in Mexico?" *Public Health Nutrition* 1–7.

PAHO (Pan American Health Organization). 2016. *Nutrient Profile Model.* Washington, DC: PAHO.

Popkin, B. M., and C. Hawkes. 2015. "Sweetening of the Global Diet, Particularly Beverages: Patterns, Trends, and Policy Responses." *Lancet Diabetes and Endocrinology* 4 (2): 174–86.

Popkin, B. M., and T. Reardon. 2018. "Obesity and the Food System Transformation in Latin America." *Obesity Reviews* 19 (8): 1028–64.

Rayner, M., P. Scarborough, and A. Kaur. 2013. "Nutrient Profiling and the Regulation of Marketing to Children: Possibilities and Pitfalls." *Appetite* 62 (March): 232–35.

Reardon, T., and J. Berdegué. 2002. "The Rapid Rise of Supermarkets in Latin America: Challenges and Opportunities for Development." *Development Policy Review* 20 (4): 317–34.

Reardon, T., C. Timmer, C. Barrett and J. Berdegué. 2003. "The Rise of Supermarkets in Africa, Asia, and Latin America." *American Journal of Agricultural Economics* 85 (5): 1140–46.

Reardon, T., C. Timmer, and B. Minten. 2012. "The Supermarket Revolution in Asia and Emerging Development Strategies to Include Small Farmers." *Proceedings of the National Academy of Sciences of the United States of America* 109 (31): 12332–37.

Reardon, T., D. Tschirley, B. Minten, S. Haggblade, S. Liverpool-Tasie, M. Dolislager, and C. Ijumba. 2015. "Transformation of African Agrifood Systems in the New Era of Rapid Urbanization and the Emergence of a Middle Class." In *Beyond a Middle Income Africa: Transforming African Economies for Sustained Growth with Rising Employment and Incomes,* edited by O. Badiane and T. Makombe. ReSAKSS Annual trends and outlook report 2014. Washington, DC: International Food Policy Research Institute (IFPRI). http://ebrary.ifpri.org/cdm/ref/collection /p15738coll2/id/130005.

Reis, R. S., D. Salvo, D. Ogilvie, E. V. Lambert, S. Goenka, R. C. Brownson, and L. P. A. S. E. Committee. 2016. "Scaling Up Physical Activity Interventions Worldwide: Stepping Up to Larger and Smarter Approaches to Get People Moving." *The Lancet* 388 (10051): 1337–48.

Rico-Campà, A., M. A. Martínez-González, I. Alvarez-Alvarez, R. de Deus Mendonça, C. de la Fuente-Arrillaga, C. Gómez-Donoso, and M. Bes-Rastrollo. 2019. "Association between Consumption of Ultra-Processed Foods and All Cause Mortality: SUN Prospective Cohort Study." *BMJ* 365: l1949.

Roberto, C. A., H. G. Lawman, M. T. LeVasseur, N. Mitra, A. Peterhans, B. Herring, and S. N. Bleich. 2019. "Association of a Beverage Tax on Sugar-Sweetened and Artificially Sweetened Beverages with Changes in Beverage Prices and Sales at Chain Retailers in a Large Urban Setting." *JAMA* 321 (18): 1799–810.

Roodenburg, A., B. Popkin, and J. Seidell. 2011. "Development of International Criteria for a Front of Package Nutrient Profiling System: International Choices Programme." *European Journal of Clinical Nutrition* 65: 1190.

Sallis, J. F., F. Bull, R. Burdett, L. D. Frank, P. Griffiths, B. Giles-Corti, and M. Stevenson. 2016. "Use of Science to Guide City Planning Policy and Practice: How to Achieve Healthy and Sustainable Future Cities." *The Lancet* 388 (10062): 2936–47.

Sallis, J. F., E. Cerin, T. L. Conway, M. A. Adams, L. D. Frank, M. Pratt, D. Salvo, J. Schipperijn, G. Smith, K. L. Cain, R. Davey, J. Kerr, P.-C. Lai, J. Mitáš, R. Reis, O. L. Sarmiento, G. Schofield, J. Troelsen, D. Van Dyck, I. De Bourdeaudhuij, and N. Owen. 2016. "Physical Activity in Relation to Urban Environments in 14 Cities Worldwide: A Cross-Sectional Study." *The Lancet* 387 (10034): 2007–17.

Sánchez-Romero, L. M., J. Penko, P. G. Coxson, A. Fernández, A. Mason, A. E. Moran, L. Ávila-Burgos, M. Odden, S. Barquera, and K. Bibbins-Domingo. 2016. "Projected Impact of Mexico's Sugar-Sweetened Beverage Tax Policy on Diabetes and Cardiovascular Disease: A Modeling Study." *PLOS Medicine* 13 (11): e1002158.

Seiler, S., A. Tuchman, and S. Yao. 2019. "The Impact of Soda Taxes: Pass-Through, Tax Avoidance, and Nutritional Effects." Working Paper 3752. Stanford Business School. https://www.gsb.stanford.edu/faculty-research/working -papers/impact-soda-taxes-pass-through-tax-avoidance-nutritional-effects.

Silver, L. D., S. W. Ng, S. Ryan-Ibarra, L. S. Taillie, M. Induni, D. R. Miles, J. M. Poti, and B. M. Popkin. 2017. "Changes in Prices, Sales, Consumer Spending, and

Beverage Consumption One Year after a Tax on Sugar-Sweetened Beverages in Berkeley, California, US: A Before-and-After Study." *PLOS Medicine* 14 (4): e1002283.

Smed, S., P. Scarborough, M. Rayner, and J. D. Jensen. 2016. "The Effects of the Danish Saturated Fat Tax on Food and Nutrient Intake and Modelled Health Outcomes: An Econometric and Comparative Risk Assessment Evaluation." *European Journal of Clinical Nutrition* 70 (6): 681.

Srour, B., L. K. Fezeu, E. Kesse-Guyot, B. Allès, C. Méjean, R. M. Andrianasolo, E. Chazelas, M. Deschasaux, S. Hercberg, and P. Galan. 2019. "Ultra-Processed Food Intake and Risk of Cardiovascular Disease: Prospective Cohort Study (NutriNet-Santé)." *BMJ* 365: l1451.

Stacey, N., A. Tugendhaft, and K. Hofman. 2017. "Sugary Beverage Taxation in South Africa: Household Expenditure, Demand System Elasticities, and Policy Implications." *Preventive Medicine* 105 (Supplement): S26–S31.

Taillie, L. S., J. A. Rivera, B. M. Popkin, and C. Batis. 2017. "Do High vs. Low Purchasers Respond Differently to a Nonessential Energy-Dense Food Tax? Two-Year Evaluation of Mexico's 8% Nonessential Food Tax." *Preventive Medicine* 105 (Supplement): S37–S42.

Tainio, M. A., J. de Nazelle, T. Götschi, S. Kahlmeier, D. Rojas-Rueda, M. J. Nieuwenhuijsen, T. H. de Sá, P. Kelly, and J. Woodcock. 2016. "Can Air Pollution Negate the Health Benefits of Cycling and Walking?" *Preventive Medicine* 87 (2016): 233–36.

Théodore, F. L., L. Tolentino-Mayo, E. Hernández-Zenil, L. Bahena, A. Velasco, B. Popkin, J. A. Rivera, and S. Barquera. 2017. "Pitfalls of the Self-Regulation of Advertisements Directed at Children on Mexican Television." *Pediatric Obesity* 12 (4): 312–19.

Townsend, R., S. M. Jaffee, Y. Hoberg-Tanimichi, A. M. Htenas, M. Shekar, Z. Hyder, M. Gautam, H. A. Kray, L. Ronchi, S. Hussain, L. K. Elder, and E. Moses. 2016. *The Future of Food: Shaping the Global Food System to Deliver Improved Nutrition and Health*. Washington, DC: World Bank.

Vartanian, L. R., M. B. Schwartz, and K. D. Brownell. 2007. "Effects of Soft Drink Consumption on Nutrition and Health: A Systematic Review and Meta-Analysis." *American Journal of Public Health* 97 (4): 667–75.

Vilar-Compte, M. 2018. *Using Sugar-Sweetened Beverage Taxes and Advertising Regulations to Combat Obesity in Mexico*. Global Delivery Initiative. Washington, DC: World Bank.

Wang, Y., L. Cai, Y. Wu, R. Wilson, C. Weston, O. Fawole, S. N. Bleich, L. J. Cheskin, N. N. Showell, B. D. Lau, D. T. Chiu, A. Zhang, and J. Segal. 2015. "What Childhood Obesity Prevention Programmes Work? A Systematic Review and Meta-Analysis." *Obesity Reviews* 16 (7): 547–65.

WCRFI (World Cancer Research Fund International). 2015. "Curbing Global Sugar Consumption: Effective Food Policy Actions to Help Promote Healthy Diets and Tackle Obesity." Brief. https://www.wcrf.org/sites/default/files/Curbing-Global-Sugar-Consumption.pdf.

———. 2019. *Building Momentum: Lessons on Implementing a Robust Front-of-Pack Food Label*. London: WCRF.

WHO (World Health Organization). 2014. *Draft Guidelines on Free Sugars Released For Public Consultation*. Geneva: WHO.

———. 2018. *ACTIVE: A Technical Package for Increasing Physical Activity*. Geneva: WHO. https://apps.who.int/iris/handle/10665/275415.

WHO Commission on Ending Childhood Obesity. 2016. *Report of the WHO Commission on Ending Childhood Obesity*. Geneva: WHO.

WHO Expert Committee. 2016. *Fiscal Policies for Diet and Prevention of Noncommunicable Diseases: Technical Meeting Report, 5–6 May 2015, Geneva, Switzerland*. WHO Technical Report. Geneva: WHO.

WHO Regional Office for Europe. 2015a. Nutrient Profile Model: 6. Copenhagen: WHO Regional Office for Europe.

———. 2015b. *Using Price Policies to Promote Healthier Diets*. Division of Noncommunicable Diseases and the Lifecourse. Nutrition Physical Activity and Obesity Programme. Brussels: WHO Regional Office for Europe.

Xia, T., Y. Zhang, S. Crabb, and P. Shah. 2013. "Cobenefits of Replacing Car Trips with Alternative Transportation: A Review of Evidence and Methodological Issues." *Journal of Environmental and Public Health* 2013: Article ID 797312. https://doi.org/10.1155/2013/797312.

6

Business Unusual: How Can Development Partners Support Countries to Fight Obesity?

Meera Shekar and Anne Marie Provo

This chapter builds on the previous chapters to provide guidance for external partners and World Bank teams working across multiple sectors on how to leverage the comparative advantage of the World Bank and other development partners to catalyze future action on this agenda. It builds on chapters 1–5, which lay out the growing problem of overweight/obesity, the rationale for public action, potential strategies/interventions to prevent overweight/obesity, and the lessons learned from these efforts to date. It links these elements together to propose a framework for how client countries and development partners such as the World Bank can use advocacy, policy, and analytical and financial tools to accelerate their contribution to the prevention of overweight/obesity.

Key Messages

- The global overweight/obesity epidemic presents a formidable challenge to human capital acquisition, national wealth accumulation in countries, and the World Bank's twin goals of ending extreme poverty and boosting shared prosperity. While investments in reducing undernutrition are at an all-time high and reductions in undernutrition are being observed globally, overweight/obesity rates are rising rapidly.

- Overweight/obesity has large impacts on national economies—both through reduced productivity and increased health care costs and because efforts to address overweight/obesity have substantial potential for climate co-benefits. Efforts to control overweight/obesity are, therefore, efforts toward building a global public good, with a strong role for governments.
- Previous chapters make a strong case for the role of governments in preventing overweight/obesity. While the role of governments remains central, development partners also have a key role, and there has been considerable discussion among partners on the rationale for preventing obesity. However, most partners have not yet maximized the opportunities to translate current knowledge into action.
- Continued economic growth among the world's low- and middle-income countries will only intensify the magnitude of the devastating impacts of overweight/obesity on health, well-being, and productivity. Furthermore, as economies grow, the burden of overweight/obesity will shift even more toward the poor, making it all the more imperative for institutions such as the World Bank to engage and to support governments in this effort.
- In its engagement with country governments, the World Bank and other development partners can highlight the issue of overweight/obesity as one that requires corrective public action rather than one of individual responsibility. And it can transform this advocacy into tangible investment opportunities. The World Bank has at its disposal a repertoire of analytical, diagnostic, policy, technical assistance, and investment tools that it can deploy to address different aspects of the overweight/obesity challenge. Other development partners have similar tools that can be deployed.
- Given the renewed focus on human capital, its links to the overweight/obesity epidemic, and the growing evidence base for double- and triple-duty actions, there is both an urgent need for action and a tremendous opportunity to prevent overweight/obesity to enhance Human Capital in countries.
- The health sector needs to lead on diagnostics, but tackling this complex agenda will require both a whole-of-government and a whole-of-development partner approach, with the agriculture, transport, macroeconomics, trade and investment, and education sectors each having a major role to play. Triple-duty actions that link to climate change offer yet another opportunity for advocacy and action at scale.
- Because the evidence base is still emerging, five key areas are identified here for further research and analysis by countries and development partners: documenting the impact of fiscal and regulatory policies and active transport and building/city design solutions in

countries where these are being applied; quantifying the climate co-benefits of investing in overweight/obesity prevention policies and programs; building the evidence base on food systems approaches to prevent overweight/obesity; engaging the private sector in each of the above areas; and quantifying the contribution of overweight/obesity to Human Capital.

- Overall, three strategic areas are identified for action: leveraging the range of policy, advocacy, and investment tools; scaling up promising interventions and policies; and continuing to build the evidence base.
- Small tweaks to work programs and budgets will not be sufficient. A transformative approach and additional financial and human resources need to be dedicated to this agenda. Building capacity among development partners as well as capacity within client countries to work across sectoral boundaries and with nontraditional partners will be crucial. Experience from tobacco suggests that this is feasible, in consultation with like-minded global and national partners such as Bloomberg Philanthropies; UN partners such as the World Health Organization (WHO), the Food and Agriculture Organization of the UN (FAO), and the United Nations Children's Fund (UNICEF); and academia and civil society.

The Role of Development Partners in Supporting Countries to Prevent Overweight/Obesity

Previous chapters have made a strong case for the role of governments in preventing overweight/obesity. While the role of governments remains central, development partners also have a key role. The World Bank Group has a corporate commitment to human capital, and overweight/obesity is implicated therein, including in the construct of the Human Capital Index (HCI; see figure 1.1). The World Bank, along with many of its development partners—including the WHO, bilateral agencies, and civil society organizations—are also fully committed to universal health coverage (UHC) and, within that commitment, the non-communicable disease (NCD) agenda. Primary prevention of overweight/obesity through fiscal policies and addressing its social determinants by strengthening health systems for the early detection and management of overweight and diet-related NCDs are implicit within these commitments. Box 6.1 lays out the key milestones in recent global dialogue on overweight/obesity prevention.

Many development partners have been engaged in overweight/obesity prevention. Table 6.1 lists some of the key partners.

BOX 6.1

Key Milestones for Scaling Up Global Efforts to Prevent Overweight/Obesity

1992 – World Declaration on Nutrition follows the FAO/WHO-convened International Conference on Nutrition in Rome. The existence of populations with excessive/unbalanced dietary intakes is acknowledged, yet "obesity" is not explicitly mentioned, and the declaration has a focus on hunger and undernutrition.

2000 – The WHO report *Obesity: Preventing and Managing the Global Epidemic* is published. Available at https://www.who.int/nutrition/publications/obesity/WHO_TRS_894/en/.

2004 – World Health Assembly endorses the Global Strategy on Diet, Physical Activity and Health.

2010 – The Scaling Up Nutrition Movement (SUN) is initiated. The World Bank, in partnership with the Bill and Melinda Gates Foundation, USAID, and the governments of Japan and Canada, convened stakeholders at the World Bank Spring Meetings to commit to the SUN movement, a renewed effort to eliminate all forms of malnutrition, subsequently launched at the UN General Assembly. The SUN movement has since garnered 60 countries as members, and nearly 3,000 civil society organizations across the globe (scalingupnutrition.org). It focuses on both undernutrition and overweight/obesity.

2013 – The 2nd *Lancet* Series on Maternal and Child Nutrition follows on the 2008 *Lancet* Series on Maternal and Child Undernutrition and includes an analysis of the burden of overweight/obesity but does not recommend key, evidence-based, and cost-effective interventions for scale up.

May 2013 – The World Health Organization Global Action Plan for the Prevention and Control of Noncommunicable Diseases (2013–2020) is endorsed. This plan includes six objectives whose implementation at the country level will support the attainment of the nine noncommunicable disease (NCD) targets by 2025, as well as facilitate the achievement of Sustainable Development Goal (SDG) 3: Good Health and Well-Being.

2013 – The World Health Assembly endorses the Global Nutrition Targets for 2025 (WHO, n.d.), including Target 4: No increase in childhood overweight.

continued next page

Box 6.1 (*continued*)

2014 – The Rome Declaration on Nutrition, a key output from the Second International Conference on Nutrition, raises the importance of addressing malnutrition in all of its forms, including undernutrition, micronutrient deficiencies, and overweight/obesity.

2015 – The Sustainable Development Goals (SDGs) are launched. These include SDG2: Zero Hunger (including an end to hunger and all forms of malnutrition) and SDG3: Good Health and Well-Being (ensuring healthy lives and promoting well-being for all at all ages with a one-third reduction of premature NCD mortality). See https://www.un.org/sustainabledevelopment/sustainable-development-goals/.

2016 – The United Nations Decade of Action on Nutrition 2016–2025 includes actions to reduce the consumption of sugars, sodium, and fats. See https://www.unscn.org/en/topics/un-decade-of-action-on-nutrition.

2017 – The WHO issues "Best Buys" and updates the menu of options presented in the Global Action Plan for the Prevention and Control of NCDs 2013–2020 with a list of best buys and other recommended interventions to address NCDs based on new evidence of cost-effectiveness.

2018 – The Third UN High-Level Meeting on Non-Communicable Diseases takes place in New York. Informed by previous meetings in 2011 and 2014 and the recommendations of the WHO Independent High-Level Commission on NCDs in *Time to Deliver* (WHO 2018), the meeting served to call on heads of state to commit to scaling up the fight against NCDs and to promote mental health and well-being.

2019 – *Lancet* EAT Commission report (EAT *Lancet* Commission 2019) highlights the role of sustainable diets that affect both obesity as well as major climate and water use effects.

2019 – *Lancet* Commission on Obesity report (LCO 2019) follows *Lancet* Obesity series of 2011 and 2015, highlights the global "syndemic" of obesity, undernutrition, and climate change and lists several double-duty and triple-duty actions to address the syndemic.

Table 6.1   Partners Engaged in Overweight/Obesity Prevention

Global stakeholders	Client country stakeholders	Private sector
Academics • *Lancet* Commission on Obesity Think tanks • World Obesity Federation • World Cancer Research Institute Multilateral agencies • OECD • WHO • UNICEF • WBG Regional development banks • ADB • AfDB • IDB • AIIB Private financiers • EAT Foundation • Bloomberg Philanthropies Global partnerships • Scaling Up Nutrition Movement • UHC2030 Civil society organizations that have played a big role in tobacco/sugar-sweetened beverage taxes and so on	• Heads of state and relevant ministries • Advocacy groups • Civil society organizations • Research groups • Parliaments/legislatures • Consumer groups	• Food and beverage companies • Public health/medical providers and their associations • Media companies • Media outlets • Social media

Note: ADB = Asian Development Bank; AfDB = African Development Bank; AIIB = Asian Infrastructure Investment Bank; IDB = Inter-American Development Bank; OECD = Organisation for Economic Co-operation and Development; UHC = universal health coverage; UNICEF = United Nations Children's Fund; WBG = World Bank Group; WHO = World Health Organization.

Preventing Overweight/Obesity Will Boost Human Capital

A healthy, well-educated population drives economic growth, poverty reduction, and future income generation (figure 6.1). Recent estimates indicate that human capital—the sum total of a population's health, skills, knowledge, experience, and habits—accounts for over two-thirds of total global wealth (estimated at US$1,143 trillion in 2018). Human capital contributes to growth as it accumulates, as it affects innovation and adaptation, and in its ability to interact with other forms of digital and hard capital to drive skill-based technological change (see box 6.2). The contribution of human capital to country wealth increases as countries climb the income ladder, with human capital constituting about 70 percent of the wealth in high-income countries and only about 40 percent in low-income ones. Unfortunately, human capital does not just appear; continued acquisition of wealth requires investments from both individuals and countries to ensure that the population has the skills and resources to be able to maximize the use of limited natural and produced capital.

With its growing concentration in low- and middle-income countries, the overweight/obesity epidemic is a formidable threat to human capital acquisition and sustained economic growth in these countries. Overweight/obesity and diet-related NCDs will directly affect adult survival; this in turn impacts adult survival rates (ASRs) and labor force productivity (see figure B6.2.1). As highlighted in chapters 2–4, the overweight/obesity epidemic will increasingly exacerbate health inequities in low- and middle-income countries, contributing to the growing divide in human capital assets between the rich and poor. Supporting countries to prevent and control overweight/obesity—and focusing on low- and middle-income economies—can further drive progress toward the World Bank's twin goals of ending extreme poverty and boosting shared prosperity.

Within this context, the World Bank has an opportunity to intervene with a unique value proposition to build human capital. Overweight/obesity is a key contributor to ASRs (see figure 6.2). The convening power of the World Bank, the financial and technical support for developing country governments, and the multisectoral engagements across health, education,

Figure 6.1   Benefits of Investing in Human Capital

▶ HUMAN CAPITAL MATTERS FOR

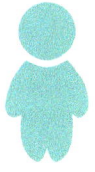

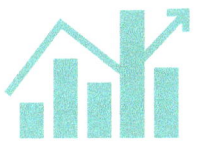

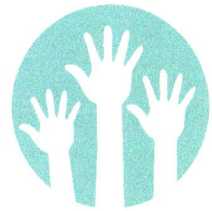

INDIVIDUALS	ECONOMIES	SOCIETIES
Investment in human capital is a dynamic process akin to investment in physical capital	Human capital is a key ingredient for higher income and growth	Education is associated with more civic participation, trust, and political awareness

BOX 6.2

What Is Human Capital and How Are Countries Engaged?

Human capital doesn't materialize on its own; it must be nurtured by the state.

— World Bank 2018

For over a decade, the World Bank has spearheaded global wealth accounting in an effort to capture the long-term health of an economy and complement gross domestic product (GDP) measures of "return on wealth." The publication *The Changing Wealth of Nations 2018* (Lange, Wodon, and Carey 2018) was the first time that human capital was included as a main ingredient in such estimates of economic progress and sustainable development. The three components of national wealth include *produced capital* (buildings, machinery, and infrastructure); *natural capital* (agricultural land, forests, protected areas, minerals, and oil, coal, and gas reserves); and *human capital* (the sum total of a population's health, skills, knowledge, experience, and habits).

Recent studies indicate that human capital alone explains between 10 and 30 percent of differences in per capita income across countries. Despite this evidence, governments typically favor investments in physical capital—roads, bridges, and other forms of infrastructure— over these "soft" investments in people.

The Human Capital Project (HCP) aims to highlight the individual, economic, and social value of investing in people and accelerate more and better investments in people globally. The HCP is a program of advocacy and knowledge work aimed at increasing awareness of and demand for interventions to build human capital in client countries and consists of three main dimensions:

1. The Human Capital Index (HCI) is an advocacy tool measuring countries' investments in the human capital of the next generation. The HCI aims to demonstrate the joint effects of health and education on the *future productivity* of children born today, benchmarking countries against *complete* education and *full* health. The HCI is built upon three main ingredients: survival, school, and health (figure B6.2.1). The last component has two subcomponents: child stunting and adult survival rates. Evidence presented in this report and elsewhere shows that overweight/obesity is closely linked to adult survival rates.

continued next page

Box 6.2 (continued)

Figure B6.2.1 Ingredients of the Human Capital Index

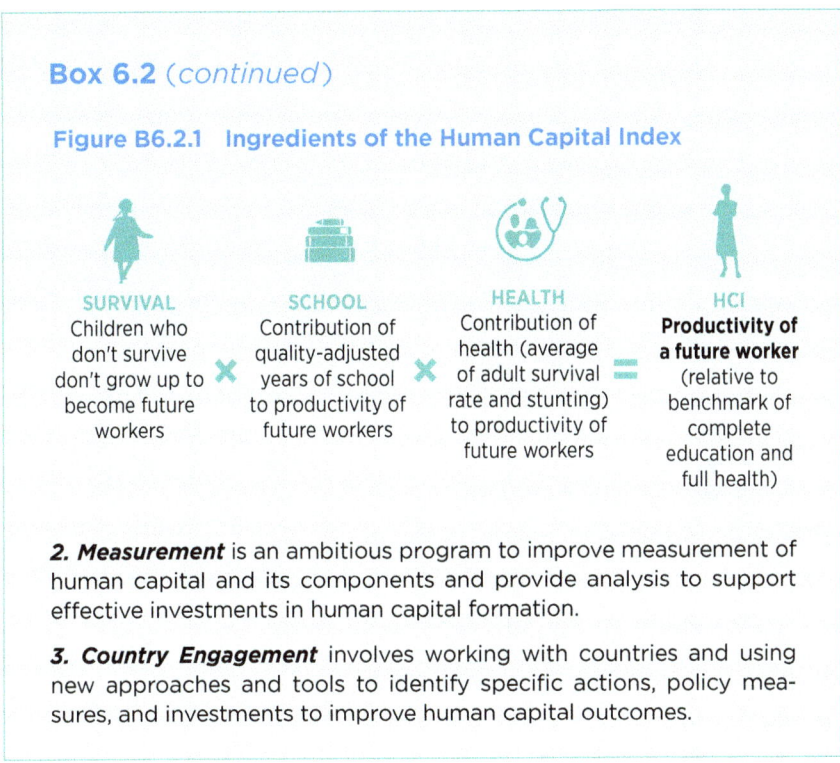

SURVIVAL		SCHOOL		HEALTH		HCI
Children who don't survive don't grow up to become future workers	×	Contribution of quality-adjusted years of school to productivity of future workers	×	Contribution of health (average of adult survival rate and stunting) to productivity of future workers	=	**Productivity of a future worker** (relative to benchmark of complete education and full health)

2. Measurement is an ambitious program to improve measurement of human capital and its components and provide analysis to support effective investments in human capital formation.

3. Country Engagement involves working with countries and using new approaches and tools to identify specific actions, policy measures, and investments to improve human capital outcomes.

Figure 6.2 Human Capital Index and Its Links to Nutrition

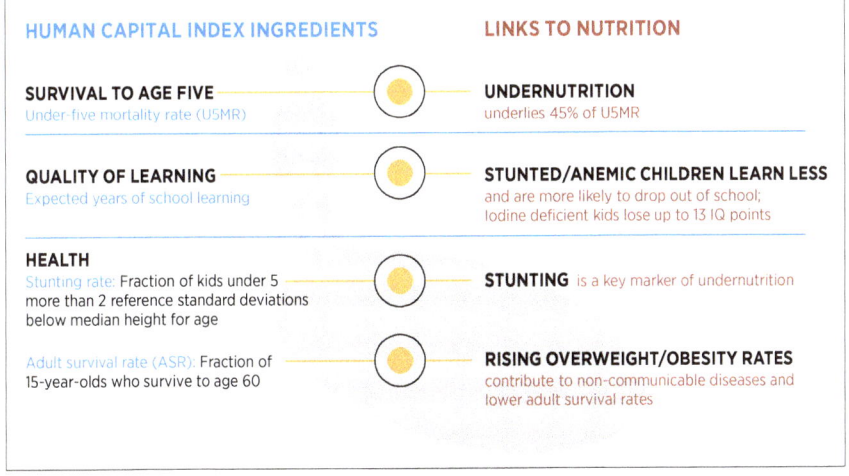

HUMAN CAPITAL INDEX INGREDIENTS

LINKS TO NUTRITION

SURVIVAL TO AGE FIVE
Under-five mortality rate (U5MR)

UNDERNUTRITION
underlies 45% of U5MR

QUALITY OF LEARNING
Expected years of school learning

STUNTED/ANEMIC CHILDREN LEARN LESS
and are more likely to drop out of school; Iodine deficient kids lose up to 13 IQ points

HEALTH
Stunting rate: Fraction of kids under 5 more than 2 reference standard deviations below median height for age

STUNTING is a key marker of undernutrition

Adult survival rate (ASR): Fraction of 15-year-olds who survive to age 60

RISING OVERWEIGHT/OBESITY RATES
contribute to non-communicable diseases and lower adult survival rates

Source: Based on World Bank 2018.

transport, urban development, and macro-fiscal sectors are unique among global health and development actors involved in overweight/obesity prevention. The World Bank also has the potential to play a strong role in building global, regional, and country partnerships that bring overweight/ obesity to the attention of ministers of finance and heads of state; to strengthen diagnostics and evidence to increase the scope and fiscal and other impact of action; and to leverage its financial and analytical services and policy instruments across all these sectors to stimulate change well beyond ministries of health. Many of these instruments have been deployed successfully for the tobacco agenda, which offers useful lessons for overweight/obesity prevention.

Besides these high-level commitments at global and regional levels, there are at least six potential and very tangible instruments at the World Bank's disposal. These range from technical support on specific issues or policies to investment lending across various sectors and to policy reforms and design of fiscal policies to deliver on this agenda. These instruments are summarized in table 6.2.

Is There Potential for Business Unusual?

Development partners have a number of important opportunities to play a transformative role in the global response to obesity prevention and control with a focus on at least three strategic areas (figure 6.3):

- Strategic Area 1: Leveraging the range of advocacy, policy, and investment tools at the global, regional, and country levels
- Strategic Area 2: Scaling up promising interventions and policies, and supporting reforms through multisectoral engagement, including in the private sector
- Strategic Area 3: Building the evidence and knowledge base across sectors

Working across these three strategic areas can build the investment and advisory pipeline with middle-income countries; support preemptive, preventive public action in low-income countries; and offer potential for stronger reimbursable advisory services (RAS) with high-income countries.

Chapter 5 highlights the promising regulatory and fiscal policies and interventions for the primary prevention of overweight/obesity, including (1) taxing unhealthy foods and subsidizing healthy foods; (2) creating nutrient profiling models and using those models for front-of-package labels to reduce consumption of ultra-processed foods and beverages; (3) limiting access to and marketing of unhealthy ultra-processed foods to children and adolescents through an array of linked regulations and

Table 6.2 An Overview of Relevant World Bank Products and Services to Support Countries

Instrument	Description	Purpose	Relevance for overweight/obesity prevention
Systematic Country Diagnostics (SCD)	A diagnostic exercise that identifies the most important constraints a country has and opportunities it can embrace to accelerate progress toward the twin goals of eliminating extreme poverty and boosting shared prosperity. Informed by analysis and multistakeholder consultation.	Informs the strategic dialogue between the World Bank Group and the client country on priority areas for engagement. Includes a thorough, systematic review of the country situation that can guide World Bank Group analytical and operational support over a three-year period.	Signals the magnitude of the overweight/obesity challenge and the economic and poverty implications to clients and World Bank Group teams/country management. Sets the foundation for further analytical engagement and operational investments in the country.
Country Partnership Framework (CPF)	The central tool guiding World Bank Group engagement at the country level. Outlines the key objectives and development results that guide World Bank Group support for the member country's development program. Informed by the SCD.	Aims to make the country-driven engagement more systematic, evidence based, selective, and focused. Defines the main development goals to be supported by the World Bank Group and a selective program of World Bank Group–supported investments across all sectors for this purpose.	Provides the space for related analytical work and lending as well as policy reforms on overweight/obesity prevention for the next three-year period.

continued next page

Table 6.2 (*continued*)

Instrument	Description	Purpose	Relevance for overweight/obesity prevention
Development Policy Financing (DPF)	Provides IDA/IBRD funds as non-earmarked general budget financing that is subject to the client's own implementation processes and systems contingent upon completing a set of policy and institutional actions or triggers—termed *prior actions*—before disbursement. Lending operations employing this instrument are commonly referred to as Development Policy Operations (DPOs).	Support clients to design and implement a program of policy and institutional reforms while providing financing to reduce fiscal deficit.	Provides financial incentives for the approval of key policies that are needed for preventing overweight/obesity. Brings critical sectoral policy bottlenecks to the attention of ministries of finance, planning, and so on; can call attention to and accelerate the process of achieving difficult policy reforms by providing policy triggers, based on which development finance is released to client countries. Can be used to design and implement taxation, regulation, subsidy reforms, and so on.
Investment Project Financing (IPF)	Provides financing through a loan, credit, grant, or project-based guarantee for a set of expenditures for a project, disbursing against agreed eligible expenditures. The World Bank Group disburses funds to the client, who is then responsible for project implementation. This is the World Bank Group's oldest and most used financing instrument.	IPF is used for specific projects with a clearly defined set of discrete activities, objectives, and results. IPF can be used in all sectors, often to build physical and social infrastructure and institutional capacity. Examples include building a road, establishing off-grid solar access, enhancing rural clinics and training health care workers, and providing micro-loans to support women's entrepreneurship in a community or region. Policy reform is not the primary objective of IPF, but a project may include technical assistance to support reform.	Can finance the policy development process. Can invest in training of sectoral staff, public communication campaigns, direct interventions such as building playgrounds or parks or bike lanes, and so on. Can invest in capacity development for institutions needed to monitor and regulate the food and other industries.

continued next page

Table 6.2 *(continued)*

Instrument	Description	Purpose	Relevance for overweight/obesity prevention
Program for Results (P4R) and Investment Project Financing with Disbursement Linked Indicators (IPF w/DLI)	A form of results-based financing that moves from a project approach toward a program approach. Disbursements are triggered both by eligible expenditures and by achievement of agreed-upon outputs, outcomes, and institutional strengthening actions defined as Disbursement Linked Indicators (DLIs), which must be tangible, transparent, and verifiable. When a DLI is achieved, the client informs the World Bank and provides evidence as agreed through a verification process. Once the World Bank Group has verified the achievement of the results, funds are disbursed.	Provides financial incentives for certain results rather than inputs. Provides greater flexibility, accountability, and ownership, as there is less World Bank micromanagement of inputs and process and greater client autonomy in problem solving.	Can be designed to incentivize capacity development to prevent obesity; or policy development, reforms, regulations, or specific outputs that trigger release of financing.
Reimbursable Advisory Services (RAS) and Non-Lending Technical Assistance (NLTA)	Non-lending activities with a clearly defined development objective that provide access to World Bank Group technical assistance for governments on a full cost recovery basis (RAS), or as preparation for a new investments (NLTA). Can range from a rapid policy note to a complex, multiyear program in design and implementation of major reforms.	RASs support clients in designing or implementing reforms, regulations, stronger policies, strengthening institutions, building capacity, informing strategies or operations when World Bank Group administrative budget or donor funding is not available. NLTA provides similar support for countries where IDA/IBRD resources are available.	RASs can provide the opportunity to engage with middle- and high-income countries to provide technical assistance for policy development and institutional strengthening, such as for sugar-sweetened beverage taxes. NLTA is usually for low-income countries.

Note: IBRD = International Bank for Reconstruction and Development; IDA = International Development Association; IPF = Investment Project Financing.

Figure 6.3 Strategic Areas for Potential Development Partners Action

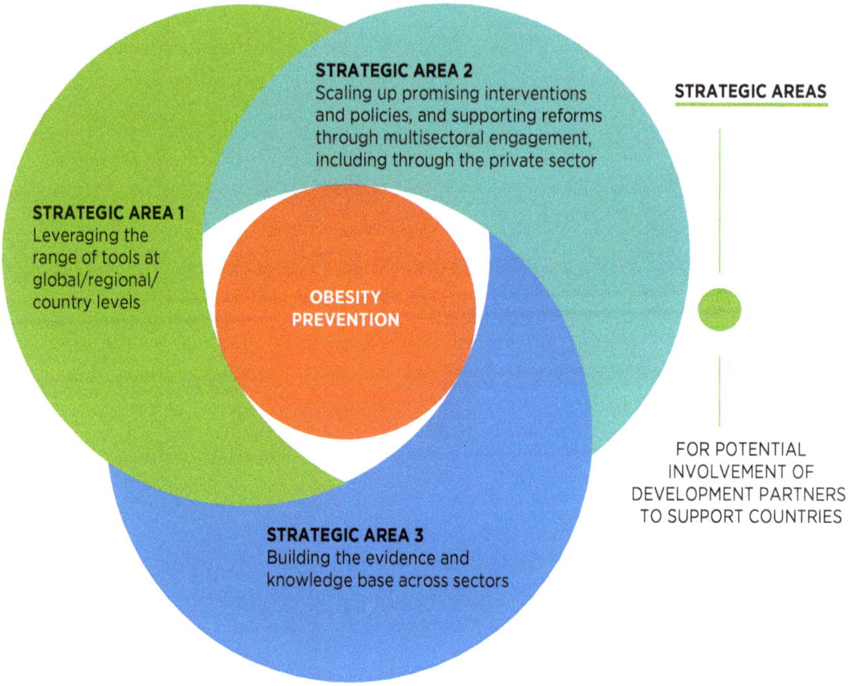

STRATEGIC AREA 2
Scaling up promising interventions and policies, and supporting reforms through multisectoral engagement, including through the private sector

STRATEGIC AREA 1
Leveraging the range of tools at global/regional/country levels

OBESITY PREVENTION

STRATEGIC AREA 3
Building the evidence and knowledge base across sectors

STRATEGIC AREAS

FOR POTENTIAL INVOLVEMENT OF DEVELOPMENT PARTNERS TO SUPPORT COUNTRIES

policies such as those exemplified by the Chilean model; (4) working with schools to enhance the nutritional quality of school food services and remove access to and sales of unhealthy foods and beverages in and near schools; (5) enhancing urban redesign and revitalization, including by promoting active transport and land and building designs that enhance physical activity; (6) promoting healthy diet and physical activity for children and adolescents; (7) increasing the quality of the food system through production, transport, processing, food environment, and food retail; and (8) scaling up prenatal and early childhood nutrition interventions. By leveraging its comparative advantages and building on the lessons learned from tobacco control, development institutions such as the World Bank have the potential to promote the scale-up of these promising approaches. However, as shown in table 6.3, this potential has yet to be maximized.

Table 6.3 Summary of World Bank Experience in Overweight/Obesity Policies and Interventions

Policy/intervention area	World Bank experience as identified through review of project documents
Tax unhealthy foods and subsidize healthy foods	• Two Development Policy Operations (Tonga and Samoa) • Prior actions for excise duties for unhealthy/sugary and salty products to improve health and nutrition and to reduce NCDs • Reimbursable Advisory Services in Saudi Arabia on obesity prevention, including sugar-sweetened beverage taxation (ongoing)
Implement front-of-package food labeling and related nutrient profile models to identify unhealthy foods and beverages	• No identified experience
Enhance school food quality in school feeding programs and in kiosks in the schools and around the schools	• Many school feeding programs exist, but these are focused primarily on hunger alleviation and improved child growth rather than on preventing overweight/obesity or increasing physical activity
Limit access to and marketing of unhealthy foods to children and adolescents	• Nine education projects that work on school canteens • Consumer knowledge and awareness appear in some World Bank engagement, though infrequently, and not specifically targeted at children
Redesign and revitalize urban areas, including promotion of active transportation modes	• Vast experience in building sidewalks, pedestrian facilities, bridges, walkways, bikeways, and bicycle paths in both the transport and urban development sectors • Most projects are in East Asia and Pacific and in Latin America and the Caribbean; four of these projects are in China • However, urban design and transport projects are not currently designed with an overweight/obesity lens
Promote healthy diet and physical activity for children and adolescents	• School health interventions are among the most common obesity prevention activities supported by World Bank operations. However, limited documentation prevents clear assessment of the content and curricula used in these interventions and the extent to which they are evidence-based and address healthy eating and healthy lifestyles.

continued next page

Table 6.3 *(continued)*

Policy/intervention area	World Bank experience as identified through review of project documents
	• Financed interventions have not been evaluated from a health/nutrition perspective • Operations financing school health span regions and income groups, though concentrated in Sub-Saharan Africa, followed by Latin America and the Caribbean and South Asia • School health projects are equally divided between education (25) and health (25) sectors • No projects focus on a school nutrition curriculum, but Turkey finances "nutrition-friendly schools"
Increase the quality of the food system through production, transport, processing, food environment, and food retail of vegetables, fruits, and legumes	• Recent projects in Sub-Saharan Africa and East Asia and Pacific have focused on increasing production and creating demand for nutrient-rich foods • There is little experience of working on retail aspects of healthy food; projects mention supermarkets but have not had meaningful engagement with the sector • One health project (Kazakhstan) provides direct support for setting food quality standards
Implement prenatal and early childhood nutrition interventions	• Considerable experience focusing on breastfeeding and early life undernutrition • Operations span regions, though most are highly concentrated in Sub-Saharan Africa and South Asia • Often in the health sector but also incorporated in projects in the social protection, labor and jobs, and agriculture sectors

Note: This table is based on a review of the World Bank's lending portfolio and interviews with key informants. During the construction of the taxonomy, a decision was made to exclude interventions focused on undernutrition, including breastfeeding and maternal weight gain. Therefore, projects supporting these interventions are not included in the summary of projects in this chapter. NCD = non-communicable disease.

Strategic Area 1: Leveraging the Range of Tools to Scale Up Investments

Chapter 5 described the range of country experience in supporting overweight/obesity prevention and control. Strategic Area 1 further identifies how these tools for advocacy, data, and diagnostics; strategic engagement; and investment lending can be maximized for this agenda. Each of these is presented below.

Advocacy, Data, and Diagnostic Tools

Institutions such as the World Bank have the convening power, along with the tools and expertise, needed to elevate the issue of overweight/obesity on the development agenda—not just with ministers of health but also with ministers of finance and heads of state. At the global level, diagnostics such as the ones presented throughout this report can bring the issue to the attention of leaders and influencers in both the public and private sectors at country and global levels. The *Lancet* Commission on Obesity (LCO 2019) and the EAT *Lancet* Commission (EAT *Lancet* Commission 2019) are a starting point in this process. Including overweight/obesity-related indicators in the Human Capital Index (HCI) is another such high-level advocacy effort. Similar analyses and advocacy are warranted at regional levels, and a careful quantification of the links between overweight/obesity, adult survival rates, and the HCI will provide further valuable information for countries. New, ongoing analytical pieces focused on urban food systems in Asia and on the processed food industry in Central America serve to fill some of these gaps, but such analyses will need to be further expanded and replicated in other regions.

At the country level, careful diagnostics can be a very powerful advocacy tool to stimulate action. For example, as observed in the Pacific (box 6.3), World Bank–supported diagnostics highlighted the crippling economic impact of the unabated rise in overweight/obesity and diet-related NCDs, showing that the annual cost of glucose test strips alone exceeded the per capita public health expenditure, with overseas dialysis threatening to bankrupt the government of Samoa in just decades (Anderson 2013). These figures shocked Pacific Island countries into taking swift action and devising a regional road map for action. This road map then served as the basis for several subsequent investment operations.

Fully integrating overweight/obesity into NCD diagnostics will further help strengthen the rationale and urgency of action, as well as ensure that as World Bank Group investments in NCDs rise, these include not just treatment of the diseases themselves but also primary prevention strategies, including a strategy for the prevention of overweight/obesity. These diagnostics can then feed into the strategic engagement process, and the Systematic Country Diagnostics and Country Partnership Frameworks can be translated into additional investments in the pipeline.

While these diagnostics can draw attention and stimulate political will, deeper analytical work will be needed in each country context to understand the drivers of overweight/obesity and identify appropriate and context-specific policy and intervention solutions. World Bank teams will need to work across sectoral boundaries to deepen their understanding of the structure of food systems, the role of food distributors and processors and retailers in driving the expansion of the processed foods subsectors, the role

BOX 6.3

From Diagnostics to Dialogue to Development Finance: Building Momentum for Scaling Up Engagement on Overweight/Obesity and Non-Communicable Diseases in the Pacific

In the Pacific, strong diagnostics, engaged country-level counterparts, and sustained management commitment have translated into growth of the lending portfolio targeting the prevention and control of overweight/obesity and the burden of non-communicable diseases (NCDs).

Diagnostics and Dialogue
In 2013, the World Bank commissioned a study aiming to stimulate country-level discussion regarding the fiscal implications of the region's NCD crisis (Anderson 2013). The diagnostics sounded the alarm of the time bomb of NCDs in the Pacific and captured the attention of the Secretariat of the Pacific Community. Subsequently, the World Bank, together with the Quintilateral Group members (Australia, New Zealand, the Secretariat of the Pacific Community, the World Health Organization) developed the NCD Roadmap for the Pacific. The Pacific Joint Forum of Economic and Health Ministers endorsed the Roadmap in 2014 as a tool to broaden and strengthen multisectoral NCD responses at the country level (SPC 2014). The UN General Assembly second high-level special session on NCDs further captured the attention of heads of state. Along with the health and economic ministers, there was widespread recognition of the urgency of the problem and commitment to implement strong actions.

Management Attention
The NCD dialogue between the World Bank and counterparts continued, and in 2016–17 the World Bank prepared Pacific Possible: a flagship program of research and dialogue focusing on long-term economic growth perspectives of Pacific Island Countries. While the program highlighted five transformative economic opportunities for the region, it also identified NCDs as one of two major threats to Pacific livelihoods. The Pacific Possible program engaged World Bank teams across disciplines and highlighted the importance of bending the NCD curve (World Bank 2017). Simultaneously, there was strong traction among management, as the East Asia Pacific Regional Vice Presidency had identified nutrition as a regional priority and endorsed the East

continued next page

Box 6.3 *(continued)*

Asia Pacific Multisectoral Strategy and Action Plan to address the double burden of malnutrition. These diagnostics influenced the World Bank's strategic engagement: the Pacific 8 Systematic Country Diagnostic included an in-depth analysis of the challenges of the overweight/obesity and NCD epidemics. Regional management further agreed to apply a "nutrition filter" on all lending in the Pacific that would aim to systematically screen and identify all proposed operations for nutrition sensitivity. With the launch of the Human Capital Project, there is sustained attention on the importance of improving diet to reduce early life undernutrition and increase healthy, productive adulthood.

Development Finance

In the six years since the program of diagnostics was initiated, there has been a substantial increase in the portfolio addressing overweight/obesity and diet-related NCDs in the Pacific region. Samoa's agriculture project and additional financing have a focus on the production and demand for nutritious foods; a project is being prepared to support the country's NCD program. Development policy operations in Tonga and Samoa have included policy triggers on taxation of unhealthy foods and beverages. In Tonga, quantitative and qualitative analyses are underway to demonstrate the impact of the taxation policy on consumption and health and to identify opportunities for policy improvement. In countries without such lending operations, Non-Lending Technical Assistance is aiming to support improvements in public financial management, service delivery, and supply chain in the health sector that can further increase the effectiveness of primary and secondary overweight/obesity prevention efforts and improve the efficiency of public resources to prevent and control overweight/obesity. Although these operations are still in the early stages, they are a positive indication that tangible results in client engagement can be achieved through collaboration and sustained momentum.

of the growing formal and informal food service sector, and the influence of markets and food environments on food choice, particularly in developing countries. Both nutrition-sensitive value chains and food environments will need to be analyzed further for substantive entry points in a manner that can influence tangible actions and investments. Furthermore, nutrition-sensitive public expenditure reviews in agriculture could also be explored more to encourage greater consideration of processed food value chains. Similar diagnostics will be needed for physical activity, regulatory processes, and other relevant areas.

The experience with tobacco control has raised the promise of leveraging fiscal policies to reduce overweight/obesity-related risk factors, such as the consumption of unhealthy foods and beverages (box 6.4). Among development institutions, the World Bank is uniquely placed to provide the technical guidance that can situate taxation reform in the overall macro-fiscal environment. To successfully advise governments on integrating taxation efforts into public health and fiscal reforms, the World Bank can provide analytical and technical advice on design issues, implementation, and strategies to manage possible challenges.

BOX 6.4

Learning from Experience in Global Tobacco Control

The World Bank Group has partnered with major global players in global health and non-communicable disease (NCD) control, such as Bloomberg Philanthropies, the Bill and Melinda Gates Foundation, the World Health Organization, and the Campaign for Tobacco-Free Kids, among others, to support global tobacco control. The World Bank Group addresses tobacco control and taxation as a development issue. With multisectoral entry points, the World Bank Group—in close partnership with ministries of finance and other related ministries—provides support for agencies with the mandate for macroeconomic, fiscal, and regulatory policy making in countries. The institution has established a strong track record of addressing tobacco control and taxation with governments and partner agencies. This box presents a summary of elements that have been instrumental to the program's success.

Resources
The World Bank's efforts on tobacco control are supported through a multidonor trust fund and World Bank budget, with a full-time dedicated team. The program has the ability to flexibly engage global, regional, and country experts to support the program's goals and policy reform, and to convene knowledge sharing and learning sessions that have moved the agenda forward.

continued next page

Box 6.4 (*continued*)

Advocacy

The World Bank Group Global Tobacco Control program has developed diverse advocacy and awareness-raising tools with dedicated resources for coordinating the policy dialogue. These include op-eds and commentaries to major mainstream and academic publications, blogs and reports, videos, infographics, panels, and conferences.

Analytics and Learning

The World Bank Group Tobacco Control program has been prolific in its publications, with country-specific diagnostics spanning all World Bank Group regions and including countries as diverse as Armenia, Belarus, Botswana, Peru, the Philippines, Sierra Leone, Turkey, and Vietnam. The diagnostics assess various dimensions of tobacco production, consumption, and taxation; these dimensions range from estimating the long-term impact of taxation on use and revenues to better understanding the impacts of tobacco industries on employment and the economy. Global public goods such as peer-to-peer learning through the Joint Learning Network for Universal Health Coverage and the development of a joint World Bank Group/International Monetary Fund Tobacco Taxation Module as part of the Tax Policy Assessment Framework have served to promote knowledge exchange across the world. Azerbaijan, Belarus, Indonesia, Moldova, Nigeria, Senegal, Sierra Leone, Ukraine, and Uzbekistan received technical assistance and inputs from the World Bank Group for policy reforms that were eventually adopted.

Investment

The resources available for advocacy, awareness, and analytics have been leveraged in order to advance the tobacco control policy agenda across the world. In the period 2016–18, six countries (Armenia, Colombia, Gabon, Moldova, Mongolia, and Montenegro) have incorporated tobacco taxation policy reforms as "prior actions" (triggers), accounting for US$1,085 million in development policy finance.

Source: World Bank 2019.

However, for these ambitions to be realized, significantly more attention will be needed to strengthen in-house technical skills in this niche area, develop models of long-term health and economic impact at country level, support countries in designing effective taxation and regulatory policies, and address the implications for food production, processing, and trade. The lessons learned in designing such policies and regulations (chapter 5) will be critical in ensuring the success of these efforts.

Strategic Engagement Tools

Engaging upstream with country clients and World Bank Country Management Units (CMUs) will increase the likelihood that the evidence and advocacy are translated into impact. The health sector can lead country teams in incorporating evidence on the epidemiology and the health and economic consequences of overweight/obesity and diet-related NCDs into human capital analyses within the systematic country diagnostic process (see the previous section on Advocacy, Data, and Diagnostic Tools). Working with country governments and the governance, macroeconomics, trade and investment sectors, the country teams can then identify opportunities to integrate meaningful activities, operations, and indicators into country engagements.

Investment Lending Instruments Tools

There is opportunity to enhance the impact of development partners in addressing overweight/obesity through tailored expansion of investments (both grants and lending) to achieve these objectives. A historical review of World Bank experience in overweight/obesity prevention and control indicates that investment lending has been the near-exclusive tool used for financing interventions to address overweight/obesity. Investment financing may best serve in low-income contexts and sectors where institutions exist and are well-functioning, and where there is a discrete set of activities to be carried out (for example, school-based physical activity). Disbursement-linked indicators can be used to catalyze the development or strengthening of often weak institutions needed for regulating and monitoring the private sector, while results-based approaches such as the Program for Results may be an effective tool in contexts where NCD prevention and control policies and strategies are in place. Given the importance of the enabling fiscal policy environment for overweight/obesity, there are also opportunities to leverage Development Policy Financing instruments and technical assistance such as through Reimbursable Advisory Services for the operationalization of taxation and regulatory policy reform.

Strategic Area 2: Scaling Up Promising Interventions and Policies

Chapter 5 identifies promising policy and intervention areas for the prevention of overweight/obesity. With greater attention and intention, investment and policy instruments can be leveraged to scale up the most promising of these approaches across client countries.

Tax Unhealthy Foods and Subsidize Healthy Foods

Fiscal policies are highlighted as being among the most promising tools for governments to create incentives to encourage healthy lifestyles, promote the consumption of healthy products, and provide disincentives for the consumption of unhealthy ones. Among development institutions, the World Bank is uniquely placed to provide the technical guidance that can situate taxation and regulatory reforms in the overall macro-fiscal environment. Moreover, development policy financing offers additional financial incentives to countries to undertake reforms that might otherwise be less politically appealing. However, to successfully integrate taxation efforts into operations (particularly Development Policy Operations), the country teams will need to build upon the diagnostics listed in the sections above to understand the long-term impacts of such policies so that policy reforms can be appropriately designed and discussed with countries. The lessons learned in designing fiscal policies listed in chapter 5 provide useful guidance in taking this opportunity forward. Table 6.4

Table 6.4   Overview of Options to Tax Unhealthy Foods and Subsidize Healthy Foods

Description of options		
Levy taxes on sugar-sweetened beverages **Levy taxes on foods high in specific nutrients/ingredients (salt, sugars, fats) or classified as "unhealthy" ultra-processed foods** **Reduce taxes or implement subsidies to increase consumption of fruits, vegetables, and legumes**	**Challenges**	
	• Strong and growing private sector opposition	• Moderate (but growing) evidence of impact (especially relative to tobacco)
	Opportunities	
	• Growing political will and consumer support, especially in high-income countries, and increased advocacy efforts	• High-income country experience as precedent for low- and middle-income countries
	Selected examples	
	• Saudi Arabia Reimbursable Advisory Services • Samoa Development Policy Operation prior action to "Introduce excise duties for sugary and salty products to improve health and nutrition outcomes and reduce the incidence of non-communicable diseases"	• Tonga Development Policy Operation prior action to "strengthen incentives to consume healthy foods"

highlights how different sectoral groups, engaging with various ministries within government, can contribute toward this agenda, using a "whole-of-government approach."

Nutrient Profiling Models and Front-of-Package Labeling Systems

The negative warning labeling system created in Chile has had a significant impact not only on food purchases and diets but potentially on long-term eating norms of children and their parents (Correa, Fierro et al. 2019). As countries strive for more systematic ways of identifying unhealthy and healthy foods, such front-of-package labeling systems may be a useful way forward. These also lend themselves readily to creating systematic cross-cutting policies across marketing controls and fiscal actions across sectors, and to leveraging several policy and investment instruments, as highlighted in table 6.5.

Table 6.5   Overview of Options for Food Labeling

Description of options

Regulate the promotion of unhealthy foods by identifying unhealthy ultra-processed foods and beverages • Front-of-package labeling • Traffic light systems • Nutrient labeling at point of sale, especially in restaurants	**Challenges**	
	• Often indirect links to traditional client counterparts • Often limited in-country technical expertise, yielding weak or nonexistent domestic institutions for regulation • Strong opposition of the food and beverage industry	• Limited World Bank Group expertise in engaging the food industry; potential conflicts of interest • Regulatory agencies often sit outside of the Ministry of Health and require inter-ministerial transfers
	Opportunities	
	• Use of a labeling system that enables across fiscal policies (taxation and subsidies), marketing and enforcement; and school health and nutrition policies	
	Selected examples	
	• Israeli food labeling program • Uruguay food labeling program • Peru food labeling program	• Chile's comprehensive ban on marketing linked with front-of-package warning labels and school bans on warning-labeled regulated foods and beverages

Limit Access to and Marketing of Unhealthy Foods, Especially to Children and Adolescents

Supporting food regulation and marketing is comparatively new for countries and development partners, including the World Bank, and there is relatively little institutional experience in this area. This is in part because these actions require engaging with food and drug administrations that are less familiar than health or agriculture sector counterparts, and very few partners or countries have extensive experience in engaging with the private sector. However, with creative thinking, partnerships, and new diagnostics, there are opportunities to engage. In Argentina, for example, World Bank support was able to extend beyond policy development and strengthen the national agency involved in food regulatory activities. The World Bank Group has also provided similar support for strengthening the capacity of such regulatory bodies in several other countries, including in India. Investments in the education sector provide entry points to engage in school food environments, both by setting standards for healthy foods provided in schools and by regulating the availability of foods in canteens and kiosks in and around schools (making healthy foods more available and unhealthy foods less available). The results of the Chilean experience with marketing regulations (see chapter 5) suggest the need to go beyond child-related marketing to a total ban during most hours of the day to be truly impactful (Correa, Reyes et al. 2019). Table 6.6 lists some of the options in this space and potential ways to take this forward.

Urban Redesign and Revitalization, Including Promotion of Active Transport

A strong and growing World Bank portfolio in urban areas—and particularly in nonmotorized transport—offers the opportunity to scale up World Bank engagement in urban environments to contribute to overweight/obesity prevention. As noted above, the transport portfolio has long been engaged in improving access to infrastructure for walking and cycling, and there are possibilities for further expanding this work to link with obesity prevention. Urbanization has changed the face of food systems and built environments, and is deeply intertwined with risk factors for overweight/obesity. There is both a need and an opportunity to consider health in community design and to ensure that building spaces and transport systems facilitate physical activity and exercise and promote access to healthy foods (table 6.7).

Moreover, local governments are often counterparts or key stakeholders for many transport operations, and there is growing evidence about the importance of engaging local and municipal authorities in multicomponent initiatives to address childhood overweight/obesity (Van Koperen et al. 2013).

Table 6.6 Overview of Options for Regulating Access to Unhealthy Foods

Description of options

Regulate the promotion of unhealthy foods, including by restricting advertising and/or media coverage for unhealthy foods, especially in and around schools **Promote healthy food choices in schools and early childhood centers** **Have unhealthy foods identified by front-of-package labeling to facilitate education of children and norm shifts**	**Challenges**	
	• Unclear links to client counterparts, weak or nonexistent domestic institutions for regulation • Strong opposition of the food and beverage industry • Limited expertise in engaging the food industry, marketing, and advertising; potential conflicts of interest	• Regulatory agencies situated outside the Ministry Health and require inter-ministerial transfers • School food kiosks serve as income-generating activities for women and alternative products would need to be provided and promoted
	Opportunities	
	• Integrate school food environment regulations into operations supporting school feeding and health curricula	• Engage parent-teacher associations and school administrations to push school food regulation
	Selected examples	
	• Chile's comprehensive ban on marketing linked with front-of-package warning labels	

Thus, there are clear opportunities for the transport and health sectors to engage together more closely to further stimulate countries' interest.

Promote a Healthy Diet and Physical Activity for Children and Adolescents

Children have the greatest opportunity to learn and succeed when they are healthy and well nourished. The education sector plays a significant role in shaping children's preferences and beliefs, and can do so with respect to health, diet, and physical activity. From this perspective, there are a variety of options for scaling up childhood overweight/obesity prevention and control efforts through the education sector. The global community's vast experience working on school health and school meals provides an entry point to engage in this space: to increase the nutritional

Table 6.7 Role of the Transport Sector in Addressing Overweight/Obesity

Description of options		
Expand infrastructure for nonmotorized and active transport choices	**Challenges**	
Encourage transit-friendly developments and compact building design	• Infrastructure will need to be accompanied by behavioral change communication or other incentives to be most impactful	
	Opportunities	
Discourage driving by having specific days and hours of limited traffic and implementing private car-free zones	• Strong and growing portfolio of nonmotorized transport projects; development of tools to support planning of low-stress nonmotorized transport networks • Dialogue about health impacts of nonmotorized transport can augment sectoral rationale of time efficiency and environmental sustainability	• Harmonize transport master plans with overweight/obesity and NCD prevention strategies
Implement workplace and school-based interventions to discourage driving and promote walking and cycling		
Ensure that playgrounds and spaces for walking, cycling, and physical activity are available and accessible	**Selected examples**	
	• CicloRutas Master Plan in Colombia	• Reimbursable Advisory Services for Bogotá and Lima on nonmotorized transport

value of the meals provided, to limit marketing of and access to ultra-processed foods, to strengthen the inclusion of evidence-based revisions to school health and physical education curricula, to engage parents and parent-teacher associations to promote healthy behaviors at home, and to create school environments that are conducive to play and physical activity. Table 6.8 highlights some options for what more could be done in the near future.

Prenatal and Early Childhood Nutrition Interventions

Healthy diet practices begin very early in life. Low birthweight babies are more prone to abdominal overweight/obesity in adulthood, and breast-feeding has a potential effect in reducing the risk of becoming overweight/obese in later life. Furthermore, improving the overall young child feeding profile and supporting improvements in sanitation and water quality can

Table 6.8   Working through the Education Sector to Reduce Overweight/Obesity

Provide healthy food in schools (healthy school breakfasts and lunches, fresh fruit and vegetable programs) Implement whole-of-school programs that include quality physical education, availability of adequate facilities, and programs to support physical activity for all children Implement curriculum standards and revisions on health, nutrition, and physical education Implement after-school or out-of-school programs promoting physical activity and healthy diets with youth and adolescents Construct playgrounds and gymnasiums	**Challenges**	
	• Very few projects support curriculum reform, which is often a political task; curriculum reform is narrowly focused on core subjects (math, science, reading), and it is difficult to influence the periphery • Little expertise and guidance are available for design of school health and nutrition programs	• Constraints in land availability for physical activity in urban schools: trade-offs between classrooms and play space • Need to engage closely with kiosk vendors to provide healthy alternatives and minimize income losses, particularly for women-owned small enterprises • Challenges exist in procurement and implementation fidelity for monitoring the quality of food in school meal programs
	Opportunities	
	• School feeding programs are often included in basic education operations and provide "low-hanging fruit" as an entry point to modify training and school nutrition guidelines • Strong evidence of effectiveness of programs in increasing physical activity especially when part of a multicomponent strategy • There is potential to remove unhealthy food from kiosks and vending machines and from sales around schools	• Most education operations engage parent-teacher associations as key stakeholders; school-based interventions are most effective when they engage these groups and other community partners, and are implemented in the long term • Modify specifications for school construction to include multifunction spaces • Early childhood development and "skills" components for unemployed youth and adolescents have promise for delivering behavior change
	Selected examples	
	• Norway subsidy for school fruit and vegetables • Haiti school lunch nutrition guidelines	• Guyana training to school cooks on hygiene, nutritious menu options

lead to healthier growth, reduced stunting, and subsequent reductions in the risk of excessive visceral fat and NCDs (table 6.9). Reducing stunting in childhood is critical to reducing abdominal overweight/obesity in adulthood and the associated risks of many NCDs.

Food Systems Interventions

Perhaps the greatest challenge (and also the greatest opportunity) will be to trigger meaningful, transformative changes in the food system to deliver safe, diversified, and healthy diets, finding the right balance of food that is healthy for the planet and for people (Htenas, Tanimichi-Hoberg, and Brown 2017; Townsend et al. 2016). Undernutrition and overnutrition share root causes in a food system that does not deliver nutritious diets in sufficient quantity or affordability relative to non-healthy options. Though food systems interventions are yet to show robust evidence of effectiveness of their impact, there is a clear need to continue to work toward improving the healthfulness of the food system and food environments (Poti et al. 2015). This involves working across the entire food chain from farmer to retailer to consumer to ensure shifts

Table 6.9 Prenatal and Early Childhood Nutrition Interventions

Description of options		
Promote breastfeeding and support the implementation of the International Code of Marketing of Breastmilk Substitutes **Promote optimal infant and young child feeding practices in health facilities, communities, and through mass media**	**Challenges**	
	• Strong private sector interests and weak regulatory bodies responsible for marketing breastmilk substitutes	• Restrictions of parental leave policy to formal jobs despite limited formality of women's jobs in low- and middle-income countries
	Opportunities	
	• Increasing focus on quality of primary health care to include breastfeeding counseling and promotion in quality standards	• Focus on human capital increases advocacy for improving early childhood nutrition and breastfeeding
	Selected examples	
	Alive & Thrive programs in Bangladesh, Ethiopia, and Vietnam	Brazil communications and maternity leave

in the relative prices of healthy versus unhealthy foods (including ultra-processed and junk foods) and beverages and to experiment with ways to focus subsidies on legumes, vegetables, and fruits as well as to control actions of this entire sector that is now inimical to a healthy diet (table 6.10). With increasing urbanization in low- and middle-income countries, greater involvement of the social protection and governance sectors may be necessary to support transformation in urban food systems.

Furthermore, the EAT *Lancet* Commission suggests five key strategies to enhance the agriculture system's impact on nutrition and the environment. These strategies and their implications for sectors involved are listed in table 6.11.

Table 6.10 Food Systems Interventions

Description of options

Encourage the production of fruits, vegetables, and pulses (for example, through alignment of research, policies, subsidies, inputs, irrigation, and technical assistance and good agricultural practices for these value chains)	**Challenges**	
	• Operational guidance and expertise on strengthening nutrition-sensitive value chains is not yet widely available	• Food processing has job creation value, and this issue needs to be addressed
Enhance demand creation, marketing, and advertising for healthy foods	**Opportunities**	
	• Healthier foods are often higher value; economic analysis of the benefits can contribute to shifting policy-maker perspectives and farmer production patterns • Small shifts in the allocation of irrigation and infrastructure can have significant impact	• Countries with multiple operational entry points have the ability to support a supply of nutritious foods and create demand • In net food importers, high-value nutritious crops provide an opportunity for import substitution
Regulate food formulation (for example, salt/sugar/trans-fat content) and/or the portion size of processed and ultra-processed foods		
Encourage food processing companies to voluntarily reformulate foods to contain less added sugar, fat, and other unhealthy ingredients		
Expand retail access to healthy foods (including through zoning policies and incentives)	**Selected examples**	
Increase the affordability of healthy foods (through vouchers and other social assistance programs, subsidies, and price promotion)	• Cambodia Agriculture Sector Diversification project prioritizes support for nutrition-sensitive value chains	• Samoa agriculture competitiveness operation links to Eat the Rainbow school nutrition campaign operation

Table 6.11 Five Key Strategies Suggested by the EAT *Lancet*
Commission: Implications for Sectors Involved

Strategy	EAT Commission recommendations	Implications for sectors and policy instruments involved
Strategy 1	Seek international and national commitment to shift toward dietary targets for planetary health	DPOs across several sectors could support this shift
Strategy 2	Reorient agricultural priorities from producing high quantities of food to producing healthy food	Agriculture investment operations will need to be designed differently to bring about this reorientation
Strategy 3	Sustainably intensify food production to increase high-quality output	Implications for fertilizer subsidies and agriculture practices in country operations
Strategy 4	Strong and coordinated governance of land and oceans	Implications for agriculture DPOs and the governance sector
Strategy 5	At least halve food losses and waste, in line with the UN Sustainable Development Goals	Implications for design of agriculture operations and private sector engagement

Note: DPO = Development Policy Operation.

Strategic Area 3: Building the Evidence and Knowledge Base across Sectors

Finally, each of the sectoral ministries has the potential and the responsibility to build the evidence base on "what works" in this emerging field as well as the knowledge base to document the "how to" of policy and program implementation. While the evidence base of effective interventions for the prevention and control of overweight/obesity is growing, institutions such as the World Bank have both a great opportunity and a responsibility to support countries to grow this base.

This is particularly true in the food systems domains, where complex systems with many players including the private sector and long impact pathways make it difficult to quantify and attribute improvements in diets and health outcomes to policy or program interventions. Similarly, few transport or urban design projects build in evaluations of their impact on physical activity, and the evidence base on the impact of taxation and regulation of unhealthy foods remains modest to date, with no published systematic reviews. Chapters 4 and 5 in this report, the recent *Lancet* Commission on Obesity, and the EAT *Lancet* reports as well as the nine country case studies produced as background documents for this report offer a growing compendium toward this goal of building a stronger knowledge base of not just what may work in different contexts, but also how these can best be implemented, and why.

The following five key areas are identified for further research and analysis by countries and development partners:

- Documenting the impact of fiscal and regulatory policies and cross-sectoral interventions in countries where these are being applied, including a focus on how these can be adapted and applied in different country contexts
- Quantifying the climate co-benefits of investing in overweight/obesity-prevention policies and programs
- Building the evidence base on food systems approaches to prevent overweight/obesity
- Engaging more strongly with the private sector
- Quantifying the contribution of overweight/obesity to adult survival rates and the Human Capital Index

Conclusions and Next Steps: The Opportunities and the Challenges

Reducing overweight/obesity is a global public good and hence a key role for governments, with support from development partners as countries commit to accelerate progress toward universal health coverage (UHC). Under this umbrella, partners such as the World Bank can step up efforts to address overweight/obesity and diet-related NCDs within health systems, increase awareness of the importance of primary prevention, and promote a whole-of-government approach to action. Action is needed across multiple sectors, including agriculture and food systems, education, social protection, transport, and macroeconomics and trade, to achieve this goal. Since many of the effective interventions to prevent overweight/obesity are multisectoral in nature, strong country buy-in is needed at the leadership level to create true multisectoral programs such as those seen in Chile. Other countries, such as Israel and Saudi Arabia, are starting to move in this direction. Helping low- and middle-income countries focus more clearly and specifically on comprehensive cross-ministry actions will require significant commitment from development partners such as the World Bank across sectors.

To achieve this goal, challenges need to be overcome. For example, the unintended consequences of a sustained focus on productivity-focused agricultural production—particularly in low- and lower-middle-income countries—have not been explicitly recognized. Despite the ongoing dialogue to address overweight/obesity through the food system, the primary incentives driving agricultural production in most developing countries aim to increase the incomes and productivity of agricultural households, improve production of staple crops, and advance agro-processing without due attention to the nutritional quality of the final outputs.

Agriculture operations are increasingly focused on engaging small and medium enterprises, many of which are agro-processors engaged in the production of unhealthy, packaged, and processed foods. Without clear guidance and alternatives, teams could continue to support such operations with unmitigated nutritional consequences. Food value chains have increasing impact on the nutrition sensitivity of food systems, with food manufacturers and retailers having a growing influence on overall diets (Popkin 2014; Popkin and Reardon 2018). Both rich and poor in low- and middle-income countries are all purchasing increasing amounts of processed and ultra-processed foods. However, support from several development partners, including the World Bank, has yet to focus on unpacking the extremely rapid changes underway in low- and middle-income country value chains, the retail sector, and food systems overall, and linking these changes to nutritional impacts through analytics or investments. Nutrition-sensitive value chains and the food environment sit at the nexus of agriculture and public health nutrition and there remains a vacuum of appropriate knowledge and skills to address these adequately. Moreover, translating such diagnostics into operations would require further technical and institutional support. The current skills mix of staff in most development institutions, including the World Bank—particularly among operational staff—is not adequate to engage on these complex issues.

Despite the dramatic increases in overweight/obesity over the last decades, and its potential impacts on human capital, this issue has not received significant attention from countries or from development partners such as the World Bank Group over the past two decades.

Historically, the most support for overweight/obesity reduction within the World Bank seems to have been through the transport sector, with some engagement in schools through the education sector. The health sector has provided little stewardship on this issue, even with the rising interest in addressing NCDs.

The renewed focus on human capital and the growing evidence base for double- and triple-duty action highlight the urgent need for countries to take action to address overweight/obesity. The growing awareness and attention also present a tremendous opportunity. Triple-duty actions that link actions on undernutrition and overweight/obesity to climate co-benefits offer yet another opportunity for piggybacking on the climate agenda, advocacy, and action at scale.

Given the need for technically sound diagnostics, the health sector needs to take the lead on the initial diagnostics, starting with global and regional diagnostics, followed by country-level analyses incorporated into Systematic Country Diagnostics and Country Partnership Frameworks. These analytics can then also feed into the wider health sectoral investments, including primary prevention of NCDs.

Delivering on this complex agenda, however, will require a cross-sectoral approach and a whole-of-government and whole-of–development partner effort. In addition to the health sector, which needs to provide overall stewardship, the agriculture, transport, macroeconomics and trade, and education sectors have major roles to play.

Paralleling the dietary mantra of "everything in moderation," development partners have not yet taken a firm stance on producers and processors of ultra-processed foods and beverages. As a result, there are competing priorities in health and agriculture with respect to food systems investments. However, taking such a hard line against health-harming products is not unprecedented: in 1991 the World Bank adopted a mandatory operational policy not to lend, invest in, or guarantee investments or loans for tobacco production, processing, or marketing. Many other partners followed suit. A similar approach for a subset of particularly harmful foods and beverages could be explored.

Small tweaks to work programs and budgets will not be sufficient. A transformative approach and additional financial and human resources need to be dedicated to this agenda, and building internal capacity as well as capacity within client countries to work across sectoral boundaries and with nontraditional partners will be crucial. The experience with tobacco suggests that this is feasible, in partnership with like-minded global and national partners such as Bloomberg Philanthropies, UN partners such as the WHO and UNICEF, and academia and civil society.

References

Anderson, I. 2013. "The Economic Costs of Noncommunicable Diseases in the Pacific Islands: A Rapid Stocktake of the Situation in Samoa, Tonga, and Vanuatu." Health, Nutrition, and Population (HNP) Discussion Paper, World Bank, Washington, DC. https://openknowledge.worldbank.org/handle/10986 /17851 License: CC BY 3.0 IGO.

Correa, T., C. Fierro, M. Reyes, F. R. Dillman Carpentier, L. Smith Taillie, and C. Corvalan. 2019. "Responses to the Chilean Law of Food Labeling and Advertising: Exploring Knowledge, Perceptions and Behaviors of Mothers of Young Children." *International Journal of Behavioral Nutrition and Physical Activity* 16 (1): 21.

Correa, T., M. Reyes, L. Smith Taillie, C. Corvalan, and F. R. Dillman Carpentier. 2019. "Changes in TV Advertising after the Implementation of the Chilean Law of Food Labeling and Advertising: Evidence from a Pre-Post Study." Unpublished. Santiago, Institute of Nutrition and Food Technology, University of Chile.

EAT *Lancet* Commission. 2019. Willett, W., J. Rockström, B. Loken, M. Springmann, T. Lang, S. Vermeulen, T. Garnett, D. Tilman, F. DeClerck, A. Wood, M. Jonell, M. Clark, L. J. Gordon, J. Fanzo, C. Hawkes, R. Zurayk, J. A. Rivera, W. De Vries, L. Majele Sibanda, A. Afshin, A. Chaudhary, M. Herrero, R. Agustina, F. Branca, A. Lartey, S. Fan, B. Crona, E. Fox, V. Bignet, M. Troell, T. Lindahl, S. Singh, S. E. Cornell, K. Srinath Reddy, S. Narain, S. Nishtar, and C. J. L. Murray. "Food in the Anthropocene: The EAT–Lancet Commission on Healthy Diets from Sustainable Food Systems." *The Lancet* 393 (10170): 447–92. https://www.thelancet.com/commissions/EAT.

Htenas, A. M., Y. Tanimichi-Hoberg, and L. Brown. 2017. *An Overview of Links between Obesity and Food Systems: Implications for the Agriculture GP Agenda.* Washington, DC: World Bank Group.

Lange, G.-M., Q. Wodon, and K. Carey. 2018. *The Changing Wealth of Nations 2018: Building a Sustainable Future.* Washington, DC: World Bank.

LCO (*Lancet* Commission on Obesity). 2019. Swinburn, B. A., V. I. Kraak, S. Allender, V. J Atkins, P. I. Baker, J. R. Bogard, H. Brinsden, A. Calvillo, O. De Schutter, R. Devarajan, M. Ezzati, S. Friel, S. Goenka, R. A. Hammond, G. Hastings, C. Hawkes, M. Herrero, P. S. Hovmand, M. Howden, L. M. Jaacks, A. B. Kapetanaki, M. Kasman, H. V. Kuhnlein, S. K. Kumanyika, B. Larijani, T. Lobstein, M. W. Long, V. K. R. Matsudo, S. D. H. Mills, G. Morgan, A. Morshed, P. M. Nece, A. Pan, D. W. Patterson, G. Sacks, M. Shekar, G. L. Simmons, W. Smit, A. Tootee, S. Vandevijvere, W. E. Waterlander, L. Wolfenden, and W. H. Dietz. 2019. "The Global Syndemic of Obesity, Undernutrition, and Climate Change: The Lancet Commission Report." *The Lancet* 393 (10173): 791–846. https://www.thelancet.com/commissions/global-syndemic.

Popkin, B. M. 2014. "Nutrition, Agriculture and the Global Food System in Low and Middle Income Countries." *Food Policy* 47: 91–96.

Popkin, B. M., and T. Reardon. 2018. "Obesity and the Food System Transformation in Latin America." *Obesity Reviews* 19 (8): 1028–64.

Poti, J. M., M. A. Mendez, S. W. Ng, and B. M. Popkin. 2015. "Is the Degree of Food Processing and Convenience Linked with the Nutritional Quality of Foods Purchased by US Households?" *American Journal of Clinical Nutrition* 99 (1): 162–71.

SPC (Secretariat of the Pacific Community). 2014. "Joint Forum Economic and Pacific Health Ministers Meeting Outcomes Statement." Honiara, Solomon Islands.

Townsend, R., S. M. Jaffee, Y. Hoberg-Tanimichi, and A. M. Htenas. 2016. *The Future of Food: Shaping the Global Food System to Deliver Improved Nutrition and Health.* Washington, DC: World Bank.

Van Koperen, T. M., S. A. Jebb, C. D. Summerbell, T. L. S. Visscher, M. Romon, J. M. Borys, and J. C. Seidell. 2013. "Obesity Prevention: Characterizing the EPODE Logic Model: Unravelling the Past and Informing the Future." *Obesity Reviews* 14: 162–70.

WHO (World Health Organization). 2014. *Global Nutrition Targets 2025: Policy Brief Series.* Geneva: World Health Organization. https://www.who.int/nutrition/publications/globaltargets2025_policybrief_overview/en/.

———. 2018. *Time to Deliver: Report of the WHO Independent High-Level Commission on Noncommunicable Diseases.* Geneva: WHO.

World Bank. 2017. *Pacific Possible: Long-Term Economic Opportunities and Challenges for Pacific Island Countries*. Washington, DC: World Bank.

———. 2018. *The Human Capital Project*. World Bank, Washington, DC. https://openknowledge.worldbank.org/handle/10986/30498. License: CC BY 3.0 IGO.

———. 2019. Global Tobacco Control Program: Selected Country Work: Tobacco Tax Policy Reforms, Analytical Reports, Videos, and Blogs. Washington, DC: World Bank. http://documents.worldbank.org/curated/en/170101548686925502/Global-Tobacco-Control-Program-Selected-Country-Work-Tobacco-Tax-Policy-Reforms-Analytical-Reports-Videos-and-Blogs.

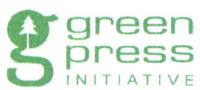